ENVISIONING A TRANSFORMED CLINICAL TRIALS ENTERPRISE IN THE UNITED STATES

ESTABLISHING AN AGENDA FOR 2020

WORKSHOP SUMMARY

Neil Weisfeld, Rebecca A. English, and Anne B. Claiborne, *Rapporteurs*

Forum on Drug Discovery, Development, and Translation

Board on Health Sciences Policy

INSTITUTE OF MEDICINE
OF THE NATIONAL ACADEMIES

THE NATIONAL ACADEMIES PRESS
Washington, D.C.
www.nap.edu

THE NATIONAL ACADEMIES PRESS   500 Fifth Street, NW   Washington, DC 20001

NOTICE: The project that is the subject of this report was approved by the Governing Board of the National Research Council, whose members are drawn from the councils of the National Academy of Sciences, the National Academy of Engineering, and the Institute of Medicine.

This study was supported by contracts between the National Academy of Sciences and Department of Health and Human Services (Contract Nos. N01-OD-4-2139 TO #158 and HHSF223001003T), American Society for Microbiology, Amgen Inc., Association of American Medical Colleges, Bristol-Myers Squibb, Burroughs Wellcome Fund, Celtic Therapeutics, LLLP, Critical Path Institute, Doris Duke Charitable Foundation, Eli Lilly & Co., FasterCures, Foundation for the NIH, Friends of Cancer Research, GlaxoSmithKline, Janssen Research & Development, LLC, Merck & Co., Inc., Novartis Pharmaceuticals Corporation, and Pfizer Inc. The views presented in this publication do not necessarily reflect the views of the organizations or agencies that provided support for the project.

International Standard Book Number-13:   978-0-309-25315-4
International Standard Book Number-10:   0-309-25315-2

Additional copies of this report are available from the National Academies Press, 500 Fifth Street, NW, Keck 360, Washington, DC 20001; (800) 624-6242 or (202) 334-3313; http://www.nap.edu/.

For more information about the Institute of Medicine, visit the IOM home page at: **www.iom.edu.**

Suggested citation: IOM (Institute of Medicine). 2012. *Envisioning a Transformed Clinical Trials Enterprise in the United States: Establishing an Agenda for 2020: Workshop Summary.* Washington, DC: The National Academies Press.

"Knowing is not enough; we must apply.
Willing is not enough; we must do."
—Goethe

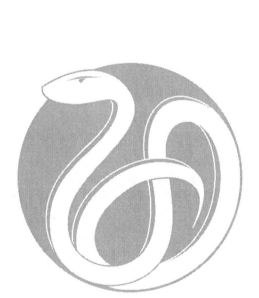

INSTITUTE OF MEDICINE
OF THE NATIONAL ACADEMIES

Advising the Nation. Improving Health.

THE NATIONAL ACADEMIES
Advisers to the Nation on Science, Engineering, and Medicine

The **National Academy of Sciences** is a private, nonprofit, self-perpetuating society of distinguished scholars engaged in scientific and engineering research, dedicated to the furtherance of science and technology and to their use for the general welfare. Upon the authority of the charter granted to it by the Congress in 1863, the Academy has a mandate that requires it to advise the federal government on scientific and technical matters. Dr. Ralph J. Cicerone is president of the National Academy of Sciences.

The **National Academy of Engineering** was established in 1964, under the charter of the National Academy of Sciences, as a parallel organization of outstanding engineers. It is autonomous in its administration and in the selection of its members, sharing with the National Academy of Sciences the responsibility for advising the federal government. The National Academy of Engineering also sponsors engineering programs aimed at meeting national needs, encourages education and research, and recognizes the superior achievements of engineers. Dr. Charles M. Vest is president of the National Academy of Engineering.

The **Institute of Medicine** was established in 1970 by the National Academy of Sciences to secure the services of eminent members of appropriate professions in the examination of policy matters pertaining to the health of the public. The Institute acts under the responsibility given to the National Academy of Sciences by its congressional charter to be an adviser to the federal government and, upon its own initiative, to identify issues of medical care, research, and education. Dr. Harvey V. Fineberg is president of the Institute of Medicine.

The **National Research Council** was organized by the National Academy of Sciences in 1916 to associate the broad community of science and technology with the Academy's purposes of furthering knowledge and advising the federal government. Functioning in accordance with general policies determined by the Academy, the Council has become the principal operating agency of both the National Academy of Sciences and the National Academy of Engineering in providing services to the government, the public, and the scientific and engineering communities. The Council is administered jointly by both Academies and the Institute of Medicine. Dr. Ralph J. Cicerone and Dr. Charles M. Vest are chair and vice chair, respectively, of the National Research Council.

www.national-academies.org

PLANNING COMMITTEE FOR THE WORKSHOP SERIES ON IMPROVING THE CLINICAL TRIAL PROCESS IN THE UNITED STATES[1]

JEFFREY M. DRAZEN (*Chair*), *New England Journal of Medicine*, Boston, MA
BARBARA ALVING,[2] National Center for Research Resources, Bethesda, MD
ANN BONHAM, Association of American Medical Colleges, Washington, DC
LINDA BRADY, National Institute of Mental Health, Bethesda, MD
ROBERT CALIFF, Duke University Medical Center, Durham, NC
SCOTT CAMPBELL,[3] Foundation for the National Institutes of Health, Bethesda, MD
GAIL H. CASSELL, Harvard Medical School (visiting), Carmel, IN
JAMES H. DOROSHOW, National Cancer Institute, Bethesda, MD
PAUL R. EISENBERG, Amgen Inc., Thousand Oaks, CA
GARY L. FILERMAN, Atlas Health Foundation, McLean, VA
GARRET A. FITZGERALD, University of Pennsylvania School of Medicine, Philadelphia
PETRA KAUFMANN, National Institute of Neurological Disorders and Stroke, Bethesda, MD
RONALD L. KRALL, University of Pennsylvania Center for Bioethics, Steamboat Springs, CO
FREDA LEWIS-HALL, Pfizer Inc., New York, NY
ELLEN SIGAL, Friends of Cancer Research, Washington, DC
JANET TOBIAS, Ikana Media and Mount Sinai School of Medicine, New York, NY
JANET WOODCOCK, Food and Drug Administration, White Oak, MD

IOM Staff

ANNE B. CLAIBORNE, Forum Director
REBECCA A. ENGLISH, Associate Program Officer
ELIZABETH F. C. TYSON, Research Associate
ANDREW M. POPE, Director, Board on Health Sciences Policy
ROBIN GUYSE, Senior Program Assistant

---

[1] Institute of Medicine planning committees are solely responsible for organizing the workshop, identifying topics, and choosing speakers. The responsibility for the published workshop summary rests with the workshop rapporteurs and the institution.

[2] Barbara Alving was with the National Center for Research Resources until September 30, 2011.

[3] Scott Campbell was with Foundation for the National Institutes of Health as of the dates of the workshop.

FORUM ON DRUG DISCOVERY, DEVELOPMENT, AND TRANSLATION[1]

JEFFREY M. DRAZEN (*Co-Chair*), *New England Journal of Medicine*, Boston, MA
STEVEN K. GALSON (*Co-Chair*), Amgen Inc., Thousand Oaks, CA
MARGARET ANDERSON, FasterCures, Washington, DC
HUGH AUCHINCLOSS, National Institute of Allergy and Infectious Diseases, Bethesda, MD
LESLIE Z. BENET, University of California-San Francisco
ANN BONHAM, Association of American Medical Colleges, Washington, DC
LINDA BRADY, National Institute of Mental Health, Bethesda, MD
ROBERT CALIFF, Duke University Medical Center, Durham, NC
C. THOMAS CASKEY, Baylor College of Medicine, Houston, TX
GAIL H. CASSELL, Harvard Medical School (visiting), Carmel, IN
PETER B. CORR, Celtic Therapeutics, LLLP, New York, NY
ANDREW M. DAHLEM, Eli Lilly & Co., Indianapolis, IN
TAMARA DARSOW, American Diabetes Association, Alexandria, VA
JAMES H. DOROSHOW, National Cancer Institute, Bethesda, MD
GARY L. FILERMAN, Atlas Health Foundation, McLean, VA
GARRET A. FITZGERALD, University of Pennsylvania School of Medicine, Philadelphia
MARK J. GOLDBERGER, Abbott, Rockville, MD
HARRY B. GREENBERG, Stanford University School of Medicine, CA
STEPHEN GROFT, National Center for Advancing Translational Sciences, Bethesda, MD
LYNN HUDSON, Critical Path Institute, Tuscon, AZ
THOMAS INSEL, National Center for Advancing Translational Sciences, Bethesda, MD
MICHAEL KATZ, March of Dimes Foundation, White Plains, NY
PETRA KAUFMANN, National Institute of Neurological Disorders and Stroke, Bethesda, MD
JACK D. KEENE, Duke University Medical Center, Durham, NC
RONALD L. KRALL, University of Pennsylvania Center for Bioethics, Steamboat Springs, CO
FREDA LEWIS-HALL, Pfizer Inc., New York, NY
MARK B. McCLELLAN, The Brookings Institution, Washington, DC
CAROL MIMURA, University of California, Berkeley

---

[1] Institute of Medicine forums and roundtables do not issue, review, or approve individual documents. The responsibility for the published workshop summary rests with the workshop rapporteurs and the institution.

ELIZABETH (BETSY) MYERS, Doris Duke Charitable Foundation, New York, NY
JOHN ORLOFF, Novartis Pharmaceuticals Corporation, East Hanover, NJ
AMY PATTERSON, National Institutes of Health, Bethesda, MD
MICHAEL ROSENBLATT, Merck & Co., Inc., Whitehouse Station, NJ
JANET SHOEMAKER, American Society for Microbiology, Washington, DC
ELLEN SIGAL, Friends of Cancer Research, Washington, DC
ELLIOTT SIGAL, Bristol-Myers Squibb, Princeton, NJ
ELLEN R. STRAHLMAN, GlaxoSmithKline, Research Triangle Park, NC
NANCY SUNG, Burroughs Wellcome Fund, Research Triangle Park, NC
JANET TOBIAS, Ikana Media and Mount Sinai School of Medicine, New York, NY
JOANNE WALDSTREICHER, Janssen Research & Development, LLC, Raritan, NJ
JANET WOODCOCK, Food and Drug Administration, White Oak, MD

IOM Staff

ANNE B. CLAIBORNE, Forum Director
RITA S. GUENTHER, Program Officer
REBECCA A. ENGLISH, Associate Program Officer
ELIZABETH F. C. TYSON, Research Associate
ANDREW M. POPE, Director, Board on Health Sciences Policy
ROBIN GUYSE, Senior Program Assistant

Reviewers

This report has been reviewed in draft form by individuals chosen for their diverse perspectives and technical expertise, in accordance with procedures approved by the National Research Council's Report Review Committee. The purpose of this independent review is to provide candid and critical comments that will assist the institution in making its published report as sound as possible and to ensure that the report meets institutional standards for objectivity, evidence, and responsiveness to the study charge. The review comments and draft manuscript remain confidential to protect the integrity of the process. We wish to thank the following individuals for their review of this report:

Deborah D. Ascheim, Department of Health Evidence and Policy and the Cardiovascular Institute, Mount Sinai School of Medicine
Ralph I. Horwitz, GlaxoSmithKline
James R. O'Dell, Rheumatoid Arthritis Investigational Network, University of Nebraska Medical Center
Deborah A. Zarin, National Library of Medicine, ClinicalTrials.gov

Although the reviewers listed above have provided many constructive comments and suggestions, they did not see the final draft of the report before its release. The review of this report was overseen by **Daniel R. Masys,** University of Washington. Appointed by the Institute of Medicine, he was responsible for making certain that an independent examination of this report was carried out in accordance with institutional procedures and that all review comments were carefully considered. Responsibility for the final content of this report rests entirely with the authors and the institution.

Contents

xi

Tables, Figures, and Boxes

TABLES

FIGURES

BOXES

Acronyms

ACO	Accountable Care Organization
AHRQ	Agency for Healthcare Research and Quality
AHSS	academic health science system
AMI	acute myocardial infarction
CDC	U.S. Centers for Disease Control and Prevention
CED	Coverage with Evidence Development
CER	comparative effectiveness research
CERN	European Organization for Nuclear Research
CF	cystic fibrosis
CMS	Centers for Medicare & Medicaid Services
CRO	contract research organization
CTE	clinical trials enterprise
CTSA	Clinical and Translational Science Award
CTTI	Clinical Trials Transformation Initiative
DoD	U.S. Department of Defense
EDC	electronic data capture
EHR	electronic health record
EMA	European Medicines Agency
FDA	U.S. Food and Drug Administration
FNIH	Foundation for the National Institutes of Health

GCP	Good Clinical Practice
GenISIS	Genomic Informatics System for Integrative Science
GMP	Good Manufacturing Practice
HCA	Hospital Corporation of America
HHS	Department of Health and Human Services
HIPAA	Health Insurance Portability and Accountability Act
HITECH	Health Information Technology for Economic and Clinical Health
HMORN	HMO (health maintenance organization) Research Network
i2b2	Informatics for Integrating Biology and the Bedside
IHS	integrated health system
IND	Investigational New Drug
INTERMACS	Interagency Registry for Mechanically Assisted Circulatory Support
IOM	Institute of Medicine
IRB	Institutional Review Board
IT	information technology
MRSA	methicillin-resistant *Staphylococcus Aureus*
NCI	National Cancer Institute
NHLBI	National Heart, Lung, and Blood Institute
NIAID	National Institute of Allergy and Infectious Diseases
NIH	National Institutes of Health
NINDS	National Institute of Neurological Disorders and Stroke
OAT	Occluded Artery Trial
PACeR	Partnership to Advance Clinical electronic Research
PCORI	Patient-Centered Outcomes Research Institute
RCT	randomized controlled trial
REDUCE-MRSA	Randomized Evaluation of Decolonization versus Universal Clearance to Eliminate-MRSA
SEMATECH	Semiconductor Manufacturing Technology consortium
VA	U.S. Department of Veterans Affairs
VINCI	VA Informatics and Computing Infrastructure

1

Introduction[1]

Recognition is growing that the clinical trials enterprise (CTE)[2] in the United States faces substantial challenges impeding the efficient and effective conduct of clinical research to support the development of new medicines and evaluate existing therapies. A gap has been identified between the desired state where medical care in the United States is provided solely based on high-quality evidence—and the reality—where we have limited ability to generate timely and practical evidence. There have increasingly been calls for transformation of the CTE in the United States to support the efficient development of breakthrough medicines and interventions and the evidence needed for health care decision making. Leaders in research and health care convened to discuss this visionary quest at a 2-day workshop held in November 2011 by the Institute of Medicine (IOM) Forum on Drug Discovery, Development, and Translation.

The workshop focused primarily on one type of clinical investigation, randomized controlled trials (RCTs) (see Sidebar at the end of Chapter 1). RCTs are traditionally pivotal studies for drug development and are often the most costly and challenging to conduct. RCTs are studies that assess

---

[1] The planning committee's role was limited to planning the workshop, and the workshop summary has been prepared by the workshop rapporteurs as a factual summary of what occurred at the workshop.

[2] The CTE is a broad term that encompasses the full spectrum of clinical trials and their applications. The CTE includes the processes, institutions, and individuals that eventually apply clinical trial findings to patient care. (See the glossary of key terms in Appendix K for additional definitions.)

both the *risks* and the *benefits* (usually the efficacy, or performance under ideal conditions) of a drug or other clinical intervention. A core premise of the workshop was that RCTs serve as the foundation of the CTE. In RCTs, responses by a group of trial participants randomly assigned to receive a drug or other intervention are compared with the progress of a similar group of trial participants who instead randomly receive the assignment of placebo or alternative treatment. To accomplish this comparison of therapeutic effects, trial participants and staff must have no input into whether they are assigned to the experimental or control group or knowledge about their assignment until after the trial is ended, except under extraordinary circumstances. The Food and Drug Administration (FDA) has traditionally required drug development firms to use RCTs to obtain new drug approvals. Workshop participants also discussed other types of investigations (such as nonrandomized trials, observational studies, and clinical effectiveness research), which, like RCTs, examine the relative success of specific drugs or other interventions and provide additional opportunities to better understand existing therapies.

In the United States, clinical trials are conducted, funded, and regulated by several important components of the health care sector. Box 1-1 identifies some of these stakeholders.

BOX 1-1[a]
Stakeholders in the U.S. Clinical Trials Enterprise

Clinical Trial Sponsors
- Federal agencies:
    National Institutes of Health (NIH)
    Agency for Healthcare Research and Quality (AHRQ)
    U.S. Department of Defense (DoD)
    U.S. Centers for Disease Control and Prevention (CDC)
    Department of Veterans Affairs (VA)
- Nongovernmental organizations that fund and/or conduct clinical trials:
    Academic institutions
    Patient advocacy groups (e.g., Cystic Fibrosis Foundation)
    Philanthropic foundations (e.g., The Bill & Melinda Gates Foundation)
- Industry (pharmaceutical, biotechnology, and medical device companies)

Clinical Trial Regulators
- Federal agencies (e.g., FDA, Centers for Medicare & Medicaid Services [CMS])
- Institutional review boards (IRBs)
- International regulatory agencies and country-specific regulatory authorities for multicenter clinical trials outside the United States

---

BOX 1-1 Continued

Clinical Trial Participants
- Organizations
    - Academic health science systems (AHSSs)[b]
    - Community-based clinical practices
    - Public and private hospitals
    - Public health departments
    - Contract research organizations (CROs)
    - Government laboratories
    - Industry
    - Private research institutes
    - Clinical research networks (e.g., Children's Oncology Group)
- Clinical investigators and research teams at clinical trial sites (see Chapter 3 for a detailed discussion of the clinical trials workforce)
- Study participants (patients and healthy volunteers who decide to participate in a clinical trial)

Primary Consumers of Clinical Trial Results
- Scientists and researchers
- Health care delivery system
- Health care purchasers and payers (e.g., Medicare, Blue Cross and Blue Shield, individual patients)
- Industry
- Patient and disease advocacy organizations
- Individual patients and families

Beneficiaries of Clinical Trial Results
- Society
- Individual patients and families

---

[a] The description of the CTE in this box is based on workshop planning committee discussions and Sung et al., 2003, Central Challenges Facing the National Clinical Research Enterprise, *JAMA* 289:1278-1287.

[b] For more information on the development of AHSSs, see Dzau et al., 2010, The Role of Academic Health Science Systems in the Transformation of Medicine, *Lancet* 375:949-953.

Taken as a whole, these interconnected stakeholders and their activities constitute the CTE. In addition to supporting the development of drugs, biologicals, and medical devices, the CTE informs quality improvement in health care and clinical decision making. The CTE is the arena where new interventions are tested under "laboratory conditions," and where existing interventions can be further evaluated for effectiveness under the standard conditions of patient care.

DEFINING THE PROBLEM

Box 1-2 outlines some of the challenges that currently jeopardize the viability and strength of the CTE in the United States.

Many of these challenges have been considered previously. For instance, the challenge of patient enrollment and retention in clinical trials is addressed in a recent summary of a Forum workshop held earlier in 2011 (IOM, 2012a). That summary describes numerous difficulties in public engagement in clinical trials, including the need for more robust information sharing among researchers, patients, and physicians about RCT opportunities; the availability of experimental treatments outside of participating in an RCT; inadequate funding mechanisms to support RCT participation; lack of prestige allocated within the medical school setting to the conduct of clinical trials; and delays and logistical problems associated with a fragmented clinical trials infrastructure[3] and health care system. The summary (IOM, 2012a) further describes possible ways to overcome these difficulties. Chapter 3 of the present report describes difficulties in engaging patients, the public, and physicians in clinical research in additional detail.

Owing to these and other difficulties, including those enumerated in Box 1-2, new RCT study designs are being developed to increase the efficiencies of trial design and the applicability of clinical trial results. Promising innovations include *adaptive designs* in which a prespecified plan defines prescribed changes to study end points and other criteria over the course of a study based on collected data and the treatment responses of prior participants; *pragmatic trials* that investigate an intervention's effectiveness in real-world conditions, rather than efficacy only (this approach may involve fewer inclusion and exclusion criteria for individuals to participate in the trial, as well as longer study timelines that seek to evaluate patient-centered outcome measures or end points); and *virtual* or *web-based clinical trials* that involve the online registration of study participants to overcome enrollment challenges posed by the current geographic distribution of clinical trial sites (IOM, 2012a). A number of workshop participants expressed the belief that adoption of these trial designs and other innovations will help to fortify the CTE.

---

[3] The clinical trials infrastructure, part of the broader clinical research enterprise, refers to the necessary resources (human capital, financial support, patient participants, information systems, regulatory pathways, and institutional commitment) and the manner in which they are organized and brought together to conduct a clinical trial. The clinical trials infrastructure is currently developed on a trial-by-trial basis, or in a sponsor-specific manner, resulting in "one-off" trials that bring together substantial resources that are subsequently disbanded. In previous and ongoing Forum discussions, many participants in Forum activities have suggested that efforts to develop a consistent and reliable clinical trials infrastructure that lived beyond the single trial could increase the efficiency and effectiveness of the entire CTE.

BOX 1-2[a]
Selected Challenges Facing the U.S. Clinical Trials Enterprise

- Increasingly high costs, lengthy delays, and inconsistencies associated with elaborate administrative procedures established by risk-averse research organizations
- Concern over lack of proportionality, clarity, or consistency in regulatory requirements and compliance protocols
- Growing competition from other countries, where research costs are lower or governments are supporting growth in their indigenous medical research industry
- Decline in the number of medical researchers, coupled with the lack of stable funding and employment
- Low rates of enrollment and retention of people in clinical trials, coupled with lackluster recruitment efforts by physicians and other providers of care, so that many planned trials are not completed
- Rigidity of the research questions that are asked, and exclusion from studies of many types of patients who might eventually benefit from the treatment (so that results of trials often are not applicable or generalizable to the typical patient population)
- Societal or individual biases toward providing potentially promising treatments to all individuals who might benefit from them, as opposed to randomizing individuals to receive or not receive the treatment in an RCT
- Inconsistent adoption of clinical trial results by health care providers, payers, and patients in making decisions regarding individual patient care

---

[a] This box provides a nonexhaustive list of some of the challenges to the CTE noted in the Discussion Papers contained in Appendixes D-G and suggested by individual workshop participants.

LINKING THE TRANSFORMATION OF THE CLINICAL TRIALS ENTERPRISE AND IMPROVING QUALITY OF CARE

The scientific process is actually part of the very basic fiber of what we do as clinicians in seeing a patient. . . . [W]hen we ask a patient what is wrong with . . . [them], we are actually identifying the problem, and when we come up with a working diagnosis, that in fact is a hypothesis, and . . . we do our physical examination and our laboratory tests as our experiment.
—Rebecca D. Jackson, The Ohio State University

Efforts to transform the U.S. CTE exist within a broader goal to develop a health care system with dramatically improved quality of care. In this improved health care system, clinicians, together with patients, families, and health professions colleagues, could formulate individual treatment plans based on interventions that have achieved the greatest degree of success with similar patients across the country and based on evidence available to support these decisions. In turn, the current patient's experiences with the chosen treatment would be added back to the body of evidence, effectively creating a learning health system that constantly builds on its experiences for the benefit of future patients.

A transition to evidence-based health care has been years in the making. For example, beginning in 2009 with its first workshop in the present series on clinical trials, the Forum has explored ways to overcome challenges in conducting clinical trials in specific disease areas, as well as in the broader population. The summary report on that workshop began: "Efficiently generating medical evidence and translating it into practice implies a 'learning health care system' in which the divide between clinical practice and research is diminished and ultimately eliminated" (IOM, 2010a). In this way, the goal of transforming the CTE exists within a broader context of clinical research and the development of a learning health system. Several IOM efforts have either emphasized (such as IOM, 2011a) or are now investigating the importance and features of a learning health system, that is, a system in which "knowledge generation is so embedded into the core of the practice of medicine that it is a natural outgrowth and product of the health care delivery process and leads to continual improvement in care."[4] The CTE is broadly recognized as a key aspect of a learning health system.

Features of a learning health system are also likely to include a focus on *comparative effectiveness research* (CER), to help patients and clinicians choose a treatment approach that is likely to work best for the specific patient; this research frontier, too, has been the subject of a continuing succession of IOM reports (IOM, 2009, 2011b). As was simply stated by one such report, "Patients should receive care based on the best available scientific evidence. Care should not vary illogically from clinician to clinician or from place to place" (IOM, 2001). Learning health system features also are likely to include use of *electronic health records* (EHRs) to accumulate data about the results of specific treatments across different types of patients. Well-built electronic records would enable health professionals to enter data about treatments into the patient record routinely. Systems technologists could then assemble treatment-specific files across all patients while purging the files of patient identifiers, and researchers could in turn mine these files to determine which treatments have worked

---

[4] This definition of a learning health system (formerly, "learning healthcare system") was developed by the IOM Roundtable on Evidence-Based Medicine (now called the Roundtable on Value and Science–Driven Health Care) (IOM, 2007).

best for which types of patients. Several workshop participants noted, however, that while use of EHRs in a learning health system would greatly enhance the timely generation of medical evidence, use of EHRs will not replace the need for well-designed RCTs.

Interest in harnessing scientific evidence for improved medical decision making and the benefit of patients has also emerged in several federal government venues. The NIH has provided leadership in the national campaign to enrich health care decisions with scientific evidence. The seminal NIH Roadmap for Medical Research, released in 2003, envisioned a nationwide system in which EHRs would be universally used to gather evidence about the results of specific treatments obtained for nearly all patients who undergo them. That roadmap has led the NIH Common Fund to support high-risk research, interdisciplinary research, and public–private partnerships (NIH, Division of Program Coordination, Planning and Strategic Initiatives, 2011). A recent presidential commission likewise advocated using EHRs to build data sets on treatment results, thereby facilitating clinical trials and other medical research—a use of health information technology (IT) that goes beyond merely supporting individual clinical decisions (Executive Office of the President, 2010). One Department of Health and Human Services (HHS) agency in particular, the AHRQ, has as its mission the improvement of the "quality, safety, efficiency, and effectiveness of health care for all Americans . . . [and] supports research that helps people make more informed decisions and improves the quality of health care services" (AHRQ, 2011). Despite efforts to forge a stronger relationship between the scientific development of medical evidence and clinical practice, much remains to be done. For example, fewer than 15 percent of the major recommendations contained in the clinical practice guidelines for infectious disease (Lee and Vielemeyer, 2011) and cardiovascular disease (Tricoci et al., 2009) are based on high-quality evidence.

PURPOSE AND STRUCTURE OF THE WORKSHOP

This Forum workshop brought together diverse stakeholders in the CTE. Held in Washington, DC, the workshop was titled "Envisioning a Transformed Clinical Trials Enterprise in the United States: Establishing an Agenda for 2020." The meeting was intended to frame the problem of how to transform the CTE and to discuss a vision that would make it efficient, effective, and fully integrated into the health care system of 2020. Box 1-3 lists the workshop task and objectives. The workshop's approximately 150 attendees were drawn primarily from the fields of biomedical and other medical research, regulatory science, pharmaceuti-

---

BOX 1-3
Workshop Task and Objectives

- Frame the problem and discuss a vision for a CTE that is efficient and effective and fully integrated into the health delivery system of 2020.
- Define how the envisioned CTE differs from the current system and suggest approaches to transform our current system into a learning system.
- Consider the following core themes in framing an agenda to effect transformation of the U.S. CTE:
  - Providing a vision for a CTE in the health care system of 2020
  - Developing a robust clinical trials workforce
  - Aligning cultural and financial incentives
  - Building an infrastructure to support a transformed CTE
- Workshop presentations and panel discussions will be supported and supplemented by Discussion Papers prepared by participants in Forum activities. Each of the four workshop sessions are prefaced by presentations from Discussion Paper authors.

---

cal research and manufacturing, health care delivery, patient advocacy, voluntary health associations, and academic medicine.

In welcoming the participants, workshop chair and Forum co-chair Jeffrey Drazen, Editor-in-Chief, *New England Journal of Medicine*, described the Forum as a "neutral venue for academic, industry, and the public sector to propose ideas for the future."

Four Discussion Papers were prepared in draft form by Forum members and participants in advance of the workshop, and they appear in a revised, finalized version in Appendixes D, E, F, and G. The draft papers served as the bases of deliberation for four corresponding plenary sessions of the workshop. The titles of the four plenary workshop sessions and the corresponding Discussion Papers were as follows:

- Session I: "Framing the Need for Change: Envisioning a Clinical Trials Enterprise in the Health Care System of 2020"[5]
- Session II: "Developing a Robust Clinical Trials Workforce"[6]
- Session III: "Aligning Cultural and Financial Incentives"[7]

---

[5] Corresponding Discussion Paper "The Clinical Trials Enterprise in the United States: A Call for Disruptive Innovation" (see Appendix D).

[6] Corresponding Discussion Paper "Developing a Robust Clinical Trials Workforce" (see Appendix E).

[7] Corresponding Discussion Paper "Transforming the Economics of Clinical Trials" (see Appendix F).

- Session IV: "Building an Infrastructure to Support a Transformed Clinical Trials Enterprise"[8]

In the workshop's final session (Session V), "Developing an Agenda for the Creation of a Transformed Clinical Trials Enterprise," the chairs of each of the plenary sessions summarized those discussions, a panel of six presenters addressed practical ways to help achieve transformation by 2020, and the panelists and workshop participants engaged in an open discussion about specific suggestions on each of the following topics:

- Suggest long-term strategic goals that can be identified and met to further transformation of the CTE.
- Describe the top three priorities for reforming the CTE based on their urgency, scope, or importance to the transformation effort.
- Consider opportunities that represent "low-hanging fruit" or are realistic short-term goals for improving the productivity and effectiveness of the U.S. CTE.
- Suggest ways that disease and patient advocacy networks, voluntary health associations, and other nonprofit organizations could contribute to, or coordinate with, efforts to build an infrastructure for clinical trials.
- Describe opportunities and strategies for developing and leveraging a workforce to support the CTE.
- Suggest the elements of an agenda essential for moving forward, by stakeholder (namely, health care delivery systems, pharmaceutical and biotechnology companies, payers, disease and patient advocacy networks, voluntary health associations, academic medical centers and universities, and regulators and federal agencies funding research).

The group discussion ended with suggestions for each of several key constituencies: researchers, the pharmaceutical and biotech industries, payers, consumer advocates, academic medical centers, and regulators.

Workshop participants expressed a broad range of opinions about the likelihood of overall success of CTE transformation. But several expressed optimism and asserted that the ambitious effort must be made. Illustrating this vision, Clyde Yancy, Chief of Cardiology, Northwestern University Feinberg School of Medicine, and Associate Director, Bluhm Cardiovascular Institute, Northwestern Memorial Hospital, said the goal is a "big solution. . . . I think if we are really talking about transforming an

---

[8] Corresponding Discussion Paper "Developing a Clinical Trials Infrastructure" (see Appendix G).

enterprise, it can't be transformed with iterative steps. There has to be some significant metamorphosis that takes place."

ORGANIZATION OF THE REPORT

This report summarizes the main points made at the workshop during both the formal presentations and the discussions among participants. Observations and recommendations made by individual participants at the workshop do not represent the formal positions of the IOM; however, they have provided valuable input to the Forum and to the IOM as both bodies deliberate on future initiatives. Presentations at the workshop addressed the following topics:

- incorporating the CTE into community clinical practice, the suggested benefits of doing so, and challenges likely to arise along the way (Chapter 2);
- enhancing interest in, and understanding of, the importance of clinical trials—from building the workforce to conduct trials, to engaging the nation to support and take part in trials (Chapter 3);
- creating a new business model for clinical trials by incorporating technologic advances and increased efficiencies and by appropriately framing regulatory issues (Chapter 4);
- designing and developing an infrastructure to support clinical trials (Chapter 5); and
- the major viewpoints expressed at the workshop and possible next steps suggested by individual workshop participants (Chapter 6).

Sidebar:
Clinical Trials and Clinical Research
in the Context of This Workshop

Although the focus of the workshop was on clinical trials to support drug development and evaluation, specifically RCTs, there was also significant discussion of the broader topic of clinical research (e.g., the use of observational data for CER and evaluations of the safety and quality of medical care). Clinical trials are a type of clinical research to evaluate the effects of one or more treatments or interventions in a group of humans—that is, the safety and efficacy of new or existing treatments (see glossary of terms at Appendix K). The workshop discussions reflected many participants' view that translating scientific discoveries into medical products involves not only the clinical trials for development of new products but also the broader clinical research methods and approaches that will guide a product's use in the clinical setting. For example, the discussion in Chapter 2 surrounding the development of a learning health system covered the role of clinical trials in clinical settings (i.e., through the use of EHRs) but also the use of observational clinical research methods to extract value from the large volume of clinical data obtained in health care delivery.

Workshop participants discussed a wide range of research methods that could engage patients and clinicians and build upon a clinical trial's determinations of safety and efficacy (i.e., can it work under ideal circumstances?) to evaluate clinical effectiveness (i.e., can it work in real world, clinical practice settings?). It was noted at the workshop that the full complement of clinical research methods will be necessary to improve our understanding of the questions that emerge through the lifecycle of a medical product. Workshop discussions included the terms clinical trials and clinical research, and this summary report uses both terms throughout as appropriate, to reflect the intention of participants speaking to the more narrow clinical trials for drug development and evaluation of existing therapies versus use of the broader term clinical research to encompass observational, non-intervention studies and other practices.

2

Integrating Community Practice
and Clinical Trials

The workshop's first session, "Framing the Need for Change: Envisioning a Clinical Trials Enterprise in the Health Care System of 2020," considered how the CTE in the United States can complement the health care system of 2020. Several speakers in this session emphasized that a CTE integrated into the future health care system would look far different from today's CTE. They outlined the case for disruptive innovation by pointing out current challenges and problems, proposed ways to link the CTE more effectively with the evolving U.S. health care system, and discussed how a transformed CTE can help build a learning health system.

A CALL FOR DISRUPTIVE INNOVATION IN
THE CLINICAL TRIALS ENTERPRISE[1]

*Participation in research is an essential dimension
of the social compact among the health care delivery
system, health care providers, the public, and
the scientific enterprises that serve them.*
*—Robert Califf, Duke University Medical Center;
Gary Filerman, Atlas Health Foundation; Richard Murray,
Merck & Co., Inc.; and Michael Rosenblatt, Merck & Co., Inc.*

---

[1] This section is based on the presentations and Discussion Paper by Robert Califf, Vice Chancellor for Clinical Research, Director of the Duke Translational Medicine Institute, Professor of Medicine in the Division of Cardiology, Duke University School of Medicine;

There has been a "widening separation" in the relationship between the CTE and the health care system, according to the Discussion Paper prepared by Robert Califf, Vice Chancellor for Clinical Research, Director of the Duke Translational Medicine Institute, and Professor of Medicine in the Division of Cardiology at the Duke University Medical Center; Gary Filerman, President, Atlas Health Foundation; Richard Murray, Head of the Global Center for Scientific Affairs, Merck & Co., Inc.; and Michael Rosenblatt, Executive Vice President and Chief Medical Officer, Merck & Co., Inc. (See "The Clinical Trials Enterprise in the United States: A Call for Disruptive Innovation" in Appendix D.) Coupled with CTE problems such as lengthy delays in mounting trials and low recruitment of patients, this divergence deprives clinicians, patients, and policy makers of scientific evidence justifying the selection of one treatment (or clinical intervention) over another.

According to the authors, the CTE appears to be neither satisfying current health care needs nor keeping pace with changes in the organization of health care. Data now available, as a result of the mandatory registration of clinical trials at the ClinicalTrials.gov website, required under recent legislation,[2] reveal that most studies are very small, enrolling fewer than 100 people, while large, industry-sponsored studies are increasingly global, or conducted "offshore," where costs are lower. Few studies address critical clinical decision points, and most take place in dedicated research centers rather than normal clinical settings. The medical community lacks definitive evidence of the relative risks and benefits of most treatments; as just one example, Califf noted that the majority of clinical guidelines for cardiovascular care are based merely on expert opinion or low-quality data (Tricoci et al., 2009). Meanwhile, health care is moving toward integrated delivery systems, lower rates of hospitalization, expanded utilization of pharmacists and other nonphysicians, and the widespread use of EHRs, the latter of which—if designed to produce useful data on outcomes across patients, and bolstered by adequate decision support—could be mined for broader clinical research efforts on the effectiveness of treatments.

The authors suggested that the transformed CTE may be perceived as consisting of four overlapping "laboratories": Innovation, Traditional Clinical Research, Health Care Delivery, and Community Engagement.

Gary Filerman, President, Atlas Health Foundation; Richard Murray, Head of the Global Center for Scientific Affairs, Merck & Co., Inc.; and Michael Rosenblatt (unable to attend workshop), Executive Vice President and Chief Medical Officer, Merck & Co., Inc. (See Appendix D for the Discussion Paper "The Clinical Trials Enterprise in the United States: A Call for Disruptive Innovation.")

[2] FDA Amendments Act of 2007, Public Law 110-85.

Table 2-1 portrays these components, which marshal the efforts of different types of stakeholders. Systemic invigoration is called for in order for each of the laboratories to reach its full potential and contribute to a CTE that informs health care decisions.

Integrated health care delivery systems—along with other research, clinical, and educational entities—should, in the authors' view, develop and implement *research business plans* in order to integrate research into

TABLE 2-1 The Four "Laboratories" of a Transformed Clinical Trials Enterprise

Laboratory	Research Goal	Usual Site	Researchers (Methods)	Participants
Innovation	Develop initial evidence about treatments and biological markers and hypotheses	Academic health and science centers and acute care settings networked with other facilities	Highly trained, with data management expertise (conduct clinical trials)	Small numbers of volunteers per trial, but many trials
Traditional Clinical Research	Determine treatment efficacy, or risks and benefits in carefully defined populations	Research centers and clinical settings	Trained researchers (conduct clinical trials and CER)	Larger numbers of volunteers, but fewer studies
Health Care Delivery	Evaluate treatment risks and benefits in the context of health care	Clinical settings	Physicians, nurses, other health professionals (CER; use of EHRs and randomization in clinical practice)	Most patients
Community Engagement	Assess strategies of disease prevention and wellness (including living with chronic disease)	Communities: voluntary health organizations, schools, churches, etc.	Community-based researchers (use patient-reported outcomes; include cluster randomization)	Ordinary citizens

SOURCE: Presentations and Discussion Paper by Califf et al., 2012. *The Clinical Trials Enterprise in the United States: A Call for Disruptive Innovation*. Discussion Paper, Institute of Medicine. (See Appendix D.)

routine clinical practice and thereby change organizational cultures and foster continuous learning. Although research technologies have advanced rapidly, cultural changes in research milieus have lagged. Adoption of research business plans, under the authority of research directors or chief medical officers, can be expected to speed cultural change in organizations.

United States-based clinical research is increasingly noncompetitive. As Figure 2-1 shows, U.S. costs per clinical trial far exceed costs in India, China, and other increasingly attractive research sites in the developing world.

Califf argued that the loss of research to other countries negatively affects not only U.S. job growth but also the utility of research findings. Studies involving foreign populations may be less applicable to the United States, because Americans may differ from citizens of other nations in both standard treatments, such as aspirin use and various drug combinations, and in the composition of subpopulations (see, e.g., Wallentin et al., 2009). Put another way, globalization, at least as it is currently unfolding, may compound the problem, already observed in the United States, that most scientific evidence is not collected in relevant clinical and cultural contexts.

The integration of patient-centered clinical research into routine health care is a disruptive innovation requiring a national catalytic agent to forge collaborations. This catalytic agent could come in the form of national leadership—several participants suggested that a gap exists in

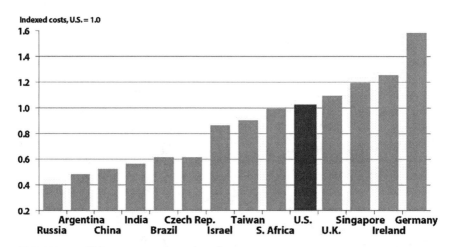

FIGURE 2-1 U.S. costs per clinical trial are noncompetitive.
SOURCE: DeVol et al., 2011. *The global biomedical industry: Preserving U.S. leadership.* http://www.milkeninstitute.org/pdf/CASMIFullReport.pdf (accessed February 9, 2012). Reprinted with permission from Milken Institute.

leadership needed to move toward integration of care and research, with many leaders in health policy and health care organization remaining on the sidelines when research is discussed in the policy setting. Bringing health care leadership and policy makers into the conversation about the future of clinical research could lead to development of a concrete, effective, and overarching national strategy.

A FRAMEWORK FOR THE CLINICAL TRIALS ENTERPRISE IN THE HEALTH CARE SYSTEM OF 2020

Controlled clinical trials are the essential cornerstone of modern evidence-based medical care and health practice.
—Robert Califf, Duke University Medical Center;
Gary Filerman, Atlas Health Foundation; Richard Murray,
Merck & Co., Inc.; and Michael Rosenblatt, Merck & Co., Inc.

In a panel discussion, the session chair, panel presenters, Discussion Paper co-authors, and audience members reacted to and built upon the ideas contained in the Discussion Paper. Participants included session chair, Alastair Wood, Professor of Medicine and Pharmacology, Weill Cornell Medical College, and Partner, Symphony Capital LLC; and panelists Neil Weissman, President of MedStar Health Research Institute, Professor of Medicine at Georgetown University School of Medicine, and Director of the Cardiovascular Core Laboratories at Washington Hospital Center, Washington, DC; and Ihor Rak, Vice President, Global Clinical Development, Neuroscience Therapy Area, AstraZeneca. This section provides an integrated summary of their remarks and should not be construed as reflecting consensus or endorsement by the workshop participants, the planning committee, the Forum, or the National Academies.

In 2020, said Wood, the CTE and health care system should serve, inform, and use each other, thereby constituting a learning system. Table 2-2 displays potentially beneficial features of both a transformed CTE and a more mature health care system. Increased productivity of the health care system is a particularly salient goal, given that productivity of the U.S. health care system fell 0.6 percent during the past two decades, while productivity in the four U.S. economic sectors of manufacturing, retail trade, finance/insurance/real estate, and professional/scientific/technical/legal services grew at rates ranging from 4.7 to 2.2 percent—and productivity of the U.S. economy overall climbed 1.7 percent (Kocher and Sahni, 2011).

One integrated delivery system, MedStar Health, is striving to develop a research orientation, described by Weissman. MedStar Health enrolls one-fifth of residents in the Baltimore-Washington, DC, area and

TABLE 2-2 Potential Features of the Clinical Trials Enterprise and Health Care System of 2020

	Clinical Trials Enterprise	Health Care System
Organization and structure in relation to health care delivery	Integration into health care system	Less fragmentation of care, as integrated delivery systems become more prominent
Objective to facilitate clinical trials	Larger, more numerous, longer, and more relevant studies	Greater use of health IT, with interoperability and standardization
Relationship between the CTE and health care system	Investigates treatment effectiveness, not just drug efficacy; treatments must show net benefit and cost-effectiveness, not just novelty	Payment driven by outcomes, not procedures; expectation that care will match evidence
Ultimate desired outcome	Efficiency	Higher productivity

SOURCE: Adapted from Wood, 2011. Presentation at IOM workshop on Envisioning a Transformed Clinical Trials Enterprise in the United States: Establishing an Agenda for 2020.

controls 9 hospitals as well as 20 other health care entities. At MedStar, research is integrated into clinical practice, with EHRs used, among other things, to recruit study participants and apply research findings to clinical decisions. Some clinicians receive enhanced payment for participating in research projects and enjoy access to MedStar's research facilities. Still, only 1 percent of approximately $4 billion in annual MedStar expenditures goes toward research, partly because the value of integrating research into practice is yet to be proved to many hospital administrators and chief medical officers, especially while hospitals are increasingly hard-pressed financially. To be convincing, proof of the value of such integration is best expressed in terms that are not only relevant to academic or health policy goals, but also relevant to a hospital or health care delivery system perspective. Furthermore, there is little incentive, even for integrated delivery systems, to use EHRs for research, when federal requirements for "meaningful use"[3] of EHRs do not mandate that EHRs include a research function.

---

[3] The Health Information Technology for Economic and Clinical Health (HITECH) Act, part of the American Recovery and Reinvestment Act of 2009, allowed CMS to provide financial incentives to health providers for the adoption and "meaningful use" of certified EHR technology. Meaningful use entails three components: (1) the use of certified EHR technology in a meaningful manner, such as e-prescribing; (2) the use of certified EHR technology for electronic exchange of health information to improve quality of health care; and

Rak expressed optimism that we are close to a tipping point for integration of research and care. He noted that the full spectrum of clinical research could be integrated with "real-world" care, and not just clinical trials. Factors supporting this optimism include

- inclusion of all major stakeholders in recent conversations about the need to incorporate evidence into clinical decisions,
- growing recognition that quality care requires scientific evidence,
- the rapid pace of scientific breakthroughs,
- growing economic incentives for gathering clinical evidence, and
- incentives for consolidation of private-sector organizations that sponsor research.

Speakers compared the United States' ability to integrate research and care with that of other countries. One comparative disadvantage faced by the United States is that its pluralistic, fragmented, and still mostly fee-for-service health care system impedes several conditions of transformation:

- implementation of a common clinical strategy across all providers, even within a single geographic market area;
- routine and smooth information exchanges among health care providers, with standard data formats;
- systematic evaluation of treatments; and
- use of global reimbursement and regulatory controls to effect change.

By contrast, countries with a unified health care system—notably, China—can apply mandates and industrial processes to create change. Another speaker cautioned, however, that although a more top-down system might be more susceptible to broad policy changes than the United States' more fragmented approach, China has many systems that do not work in practice and may not be a model to emulate.

Some workshop participants discussed the challenge of recruiting clinicians to participate directly in the development and implementation of a clinical trial as an investigator or refer their patients to clinical trials:

- There are many challenges associated with use of Medicare funds for research in clinical settings. Moreover, congressional resistance

---

(3) the use of certified EHR technology to submit clinical quality and other measures. For more information, visit https://www.cms.gov/EHRIncentivePrograms/30_Meaningful_Use.asp (accessed March 28, 2012).

to using research results for reimbursement purposes has emerged. The political controversy could limit the potential utility of findings obtained through studies sponsored by the new, comparative effectiveness–oriented Patient-Centered Outcomes Research Institute (PCORI).

- Many clinicians who might be interested in research are otherwise being compelled to increase clinical productivity and so may be less receptive to additional demands on their time.
- Cultural barriers have also been identified, to the extent that clinicians may not welcome research findings that cast doubt on the effectiveness of procedures that make up a substantial portion of their practices. Califf and Wood suggested that negative research results often are not used by practitioners; for example, it is questionable whether most physicians treating dyspnea in patients with acute heart failure are changing their prescribing patterns to conform with results of a recent study that concluded that nesiritide cannot be recommended for early relief of dyspnea for the broad population of patients with acute heart failure (O'Connor et al., 2011; see also Topol, 2005).
- Medical schools and students tend to see research as a separate track from clinical practice (although some schools now require students to conduct a research project). Box 2-1 displays these and other aspects of the challenge of persuading clinicians to contribute to research efforts, as noted by individual workshop participants.

To build momentum for change in this environment, a participant suggested, success stories, or "small wins," are needed, for example, progress in interoperability or data standardization. Oncologists were described as pointing the way toward a future of smaller, faster, more targeted trials, accompanied by genetic screening. Similarly, New York State's Partnership to Advance Clinical electronic Research (PACeR) was described as an example of an industry–academic collaborative established to use EHR data on a continuing, sustainable basis. Many of the comments included the observation that a cultural shift is called for to achieve transformative change. One participant stated

> that cultural shift has to be that it is unacceptable for a patient encounter to occur without a question being asked about whether this patient at this point in time can contribute to our bigger knowledge, our greater knowledge about health care.

BOX 2-1[a]
Some Aspects of the Challenge of
Persuading Clinicians to Engage in Research

Issues Affecting Clinician Incentives to Enroll Patients
- Lack of demand from patients to participate in research
- Inadequate, unsystematic methods of informing clinicians about ongoing or new research studies and clinical trials
- Information overload; a physician might receive hundreds of emails per day concerning clinical trials but none coming from an entity or individual the physician knows or trusts
- If a clinician is not participating in the trial as an investigator, there is concern over the failure of communication with researchers throughout the lifecycle of a study, including concern by clinicians that they will be unaware of treatments and side effects their patients experience as part of the study
- Need for consideration of patients' insurance coverage, or lack thereof, which could determine whether a research study would make financial sense for a patient under a particular clinician's care
- Heterogeneous patient mix and a diversity of patient medical needs that may or may not be solved or improved through care received in a research study

Issues Affecting Clinician Willingness to Incorporate Clinical Research into Their Clinical Practice
- Absence of cultural awareness and commitment to the principle that physician-patient encounters should generally contribute to the body of scientific evidence
- Rising productivity pressures and other demands on physicians' time
- Prospective income loss for physicians performing procedures that are found ineffective
- Lack of reimbursement incentives by Medicare and other third-party payers for physicians to devote time to clinical research, including clinical trials
- Patient information in a physician's office is collected both for direct patient care purposes and to support administrative claims requirements. In many cases, new IT tools and increased staff time will be needed to collect the additional information necessary for a research study

Issues Affecting Clinician Use of Medical Evidence in Decision Making
- Medical schools' separation of research from practice
- Lack of clinician knowledge as to the array of clinical trials available and how participation in a research study might benefit their patients

---

[a] This box provides a list of suggestions from the workshop audience, themes contained in a summary of the previous IOM workshop on clinical trials and public engagement (IOM, 2012a), and speaker presentations by Alastair Wood, Professor of Medicine and Pharmacology, Weill Cornell Medical College, and Partner, Symphony Capital LLC; Neil Weissman, President of MedStar Health Research Institute, Professor of Medicine at Georgetown University School of Medicine, and Director of the Cardiovascular Core Laboratories at Washington Hospital Center, Washington, DC; and Ihor Rak, Vice President, Global Clinical Development, Neuroscience Therapy Area, AstraZeneca.

THE LEARNING HEALTH SYSTEM[4]

*We seek the development of a learning health system which
generates and applies the best evidence for the collaborative health
care choices of each patient and provider; drives the process of
discovery as a natural outgrowth of patient care; and ensures
innovation, quality, safety, and value in health care.*
—*IOM Roundtable on Value and Science-Driven Health Care,
Roundtable Charter*[5]

There is abundant reason to be sanguine about the prospects for transformation of the CTE, said Richard Platt, Professor and Chair of the Department of Population Medicine at Harvard Medical School and Executive Director of the Harvard Pilgrim Health Care Institute, because this requires not only developing but, equally important, *applying* scientific evidence. According to Platt, participants in the IOM's Roundtable on Value and Science-Driven Health Care seek a health care system in which 9 of every 10 clinical decisions are evidence based by 2020. Roundtable efforts include five Innovation Collaboratives: Best Practices, Value Incentives, Evidence Communication, Clinical Effectiveness Research, and Digital Learning. The Roundtable has recognized in meetings and reports that evidence-based clinical decision making depends on the establishment of a health system that learns both what care to deliver and how to deliver it. This knowledge can be developed through the secondary use of clinical data, provided there is adequate governance and coordination of health information.

Multiple public–private partnerships are building platforms for secondary use of clinical data, Platt noted. First, the Office of the National Coordinator for Health Information Technology has launched a Query Health initiative—an effort to distribute "population health queries." As envisioned, researchers' and health care providers' requests for information about health care outcomes in large populations will be answered with information assembled from EHRs and other data sets maintained by integrated delivery systems and other sources. In voluntarily sharing their data in response to a query, health care organizations maintain control of their data behind their firewalls, allowing them to maintain security and

---

[4] This section is based on a keynote address by Richard Platt, Professor and Chair of the Department of Population Medicine at Harvard Medical School and Executive Director of the Harvard Pilgrim Health Care Institute; and on the speaker presentations of Bryan Luce, Senior Vice President for Science Policy, United BioSource Corporation; and Peter Yu, Director of Cancer Research, Palo Alto Medical Foundation.

[5] For additional information on the work of the Roundtable, visit http://iom.edu/Activities/Quality/VSRT.aspx (accessed March 28, 2012).

patient privacy. This and similar approaches require a standard clinical information model, such as Informatics for Integrating Biology and the Bedside (i2b2).[6] Second, the FDA's Mini-Sentinel distributed database initiative is exploring ways to develop evidence about the postmarketing safety of drugs, vaccines, and other products through data obtained from multiple sources.[7] As of July 2011, Mini-Sentinel contains quality-checked data from 17 partner organizations, mostly large insurers and integrated delivery systems, covering nearly 100 million people (Platt et al., 2012). Its features include an operations center, secure portal, and opportunities by the partners to examine the queries that are distributed and review their own results before submitting them for pooling with results from other partners.

Third and perhaps most significant, CER is gaining strength. Currently, only 0.1 percent of health expenditures are devoted to this important research and development activity, but it is expanding. Steps involved in building a mature CER system might include the following:

- *Build the research base*—weave CER into the fabric of care, so that clinicians do not have to choose to participate or perform extra steps in its conduct;
- *Build the business case*—align financial incentives for providers with quality of care;
- *Address regulatory barriers*—relax or harmonize requirements for informed consent, patient privacy, and other mandated protections, when appropriate;
- *Align quality improvement with CER*—embed both approaches into the routine delivery of care to help produce a learning health system; and
- *Build demand for scientific evidence from patients, providers, payers, and purchasers*—involve everyone in the transformation.

An example of effective collaboration in CER is the Hospital Corporation of America (HCA)-based, 42-hospital, 75,000-patient study of methicillin-resistant *Staphylococcus Aureus* (MRSA), the highly antibiotic-resistant pathogen affecting hospitals nationwide (Platt et al., 2010). The study, called REDUCE (Randomized Evaluation of Decolonization versus Universal Clearance to Eliminate)-MRSA, is comparing routine decoloni-

---

[6] Informatics for Integrating Biology and the Bedside (i2b2), developed by the NIH-supported National Center for Biomedical Computing based at Partners HealthCare System (i2b2, 2011).

[7] Mini-Sentinel is a pilot program for the FDA's more extensive Sentinel System, now being developed in response to provisions of the Federal Food and Drug Amendments Act of 2007.

zation of critical care patients with contact precautions to evaluate the best way to prevent MRSA and its spread. The study's cluster (hospital-level) randomization approach, a central IRB, centralized informatics, and a unified data warehouse help keep cost and time commitments down. In addition, HCA's corporate leadership is committed and the hospitals' quality assurance staff and infection control practitioners are lending significant expertise and staff time to the study, precluding the need for traditional clinical monitors or dedicated staff. The study was funded with approximately $1 million from HCA and $2 million from federal agencies. HCA is in a position to apply the results consistently throughout its entire system, so the study in effect offers the advantage of determining both efficacy and effectiveness. Platt suggested that the successful marriage of research and delivery of care in this example of a collaborative CER study shows that a business case exists for answering important questions of interest to the health care system.

Bryan Luce, Senior Vice President for Science Policy, United BioSource Corporation, suggested a potentially transformative "learn and confirm" strategy for seamlessly integrating traditional clinical trials for drug development and the generation of evidence to guide clinical guidelines and coverage and reimbursement decisions for a health product. Under this strategy, manufacturers partner with health plans and integrated health systems (IHSs) to engage in a dynamic, adaptive clinical trial process that begins with a tightly controlled RCT that increasingly expands the inclusion criteria for the trial so that eventually the study population approximates the usual care setting. The discreet phases of drug development (Phase I-IV clinical trials) are replaced by an adaptive trial design that facilitates the generation of real-world medical evidence as a product builds toward being available on the market. Potential advantages of this more flexible research strategy include faster and cheaper development of drugs, evidence-based clinical decisions, and payment only for uses that are generally safe and are effective in the relevant population. Registration of a product can take place much earlier and be coordinated with coverage and payment decisions, evidence standards, and thresholds.

The use of adaptive designs and other pragmatic approaches, such as cluster trial designs and virtual trial designs, was also illustrated by Peter Yu, Director of Cancer Research, Palo Alto Medical Foundation. Traditional clinical trials ignore participants who don't respond to the study drug being tested, Yu explained. However, a sequential trial design can accommodate investigation of multiple drugs, administered in a tiered fashion that allows the initial nonresponder study participant to receive other treatments that might work for them (Figure 2-2).

These more flexible strategies allow for learning from every patient, including nonresponders, about the molecular basis of disease. According

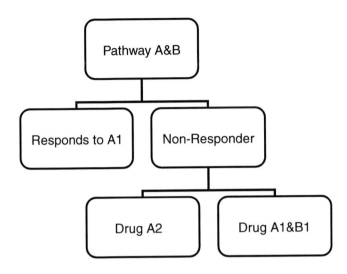

FIGURE 2-2 Example of a sequential clinical trial design that administers and tests three drugs (drug A1, A2 and B1) in a tiered fashion.
SOURCE: Yu, 2011. Presentation at IOM workshop on Envisioning a Transformed Clinical Trials Enterprise in the United States: Establishing an Agenda for 2020.

to Yu, these designs will pave the way to advance personalized medicine, in which interventions are tailored to patients based on biologic markers and other individual traits. The strategies also promote a learning system. It is important to investigate primarily those clinical questions for which potential drug prescribers and users—clinicians and patients—actually want answers, or else the research effort will be wasted. In this targeted way, and because more advanced trial designs are expected to result in a trial failure rate well below today's level of about 85 percent, a learning system is also a "lean" system.

3

Improving Public Participation in Clinical Trials

In previous Forum workshops in the clinical trials series (IOM, 2010a, 2012a), it has been repeatedly observed that increased public understanding of, and commitment to, the importance of clinical trials is a key component of enhancing the CTE and achieving a learning health system. The participation of both clinicians and patients and healthy volunteers has been considered in these discussions. The workshop's second session, "Developing a Robust Clinical Trials Workforce," and the following keynote session explored ways to identify and meet workforce needs and to enhance public engagement in the CTE. Many speakers noted that there is an insufficient supply of highly trained researchers to lead, conduct, and analyze clinical trials and proposed how a shortfall of these professionals might be overcome. Building on discussions from a previous IOM workshop (IOM, 2012a), participants further elaborated on ways to expand people's support for, and involvement in, clinical trials.

DEVELOPING A ROBUST CLINICAL TRIALS WORKFORCE

Should we go so far as to expect, not just encourage,
participation in research?
—Ann Bonham, Association of American Medical Colleges;
Robert Califf, Duke University Medical Center;
Elaine Gallin, QE Philanthropic Advisors; and
Michael Lauer, National Heart, Lung, and Blood Institute (NHLBI)

A Five-Tiered Structure[1]

A clinical trials workforce, organized in several dimensions that reflect the broad mission of the CTE, the specific disciplines involved, and the levels of desirable expertise, would consist of several overlapping groups. A construct of five workforce groups was described in a Discussion Paper prepared by Ann Bonham, Chief Scientific Officer, Association of American Medical Colleges; Robert Califf, Duke University Medical Center; Elaine Gallin, Principal, QE Philanthropic Advisors; and Michael Lauer, Director, Division of Cardiovascular Sciences, National Heart, Lung, and Blood Institute (NHLBI), NIH. (See "Developing a Robust Clinical Trials Workforce" in Appendix E.) The co-authors suggested that the structure of the workforce groups necessary to meet the demands of the CTE might resemble a pyramid with five tiers (see Figure 3-1):

- *Public*—the broadest base of the pyramid consists of patients, families, and citizens who, in the final analysis, have the greatest stake in research results. This tier consists of engaged citizens who support development of the CTE as a national resource or public good and who enroll in trials on a volunteer or basis.
- *Community practitioners*—health professionals who participate in trials as part of their clinical practices, or at least help enroll their patients as participants. This group will include physicians, nurses, pharmacists, social workers, physical therapists, respiratory therapists, and other health professionals.
- *Implementers*—individuals who devote specified portions of their professional efforts to serving as principal investigators or collaborating co-investigators, with primary responsibility for implementing clinical trials at a hospital or research site. This workforce group would include physician-scientists, nurse-investigators, clinical pharmacologists, research-oriented social workers, operations specialists, data managers, computer specialists, clinical research coordinators, and research site managers.
- *Investigators*—leaders and designers of clinical trials and scientific experts who develop tools and innovative approaches for conduct-

---

[1] This section is based on the presentations and Discussion Paper by Ann Bonham, Chief Scientific Officer, Association of American Medical Colleges (unable to attend workshop); Robert Califf, Vice Chancellor for Clinical Research, Director of the Duke Translational Medicine Institute, and Professor of Medicine in the Division of Cardiology at the Duke University Medical Center; Elaine Gallin, Principal, QE Philanthropic Advisors; and Michael Lauer, Director, Division of Cardiovascular Sciences, National Heart, Lung, and Blood Institute (NHLBI), NIH. (See Appendix E for the Discussion Paper "Developing a Robust Clinical Trials Workforce.")

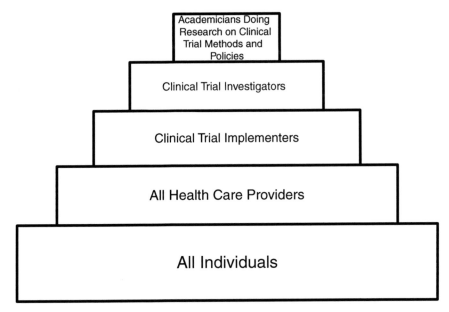

FIGURE 3-1 Five suggested tiers for the workforce to meet the demands of a transformed clinical trials enterprise.
SOURCE: Bonham et al, 2012. *Developing a Robust Clinical Trials Workforce*. Discussion Paper, Institute of Medicine. (See Appendix E.)

ing trials. This group will include biostatisticians and informaticists, among others.

- *Methodologists*—the apex of the pyramid consists of research-minded experts who explore the methodologies of conducting clinical trials and design the analysis portions of studies. This group of academicians will include clinical investigators, biostatisticians, epidemiologists, and health services researchers.

The co-authors postulated that a great deal of mobility and teamwork would occur among and across these groups. Each tier, in this vision, would be associated with appropriate education or training, geared to individuals' interests and capabilities. This would include training in research cooperation, or teamwork, across disciplines and among workforce groups. Table 3-1 suggests how other training essentials might match up with the five described tiers. In general, according to the co-authors, the size of each tier is currently inadequate to contribute enough knowledge to achieve transformation of the CTE. Expanding the size of the three top tiers (methodologists, investigators, and implementers) could require development of more rewarding career paths.

TABLE 3-1 Education and Training Needs of Groups in the Clinical Trials Workforce

Workforce Group[a]	Education and Training Needs
Public	Awareness of how clinical research can lead to higher quality care; information about available trials and concept of equipoise[b]; relevant informed consent policies. Marketing techniques might be used to reach this group.
Community Practitioners	Introduction to clinical trials; core competencies in translational and clinical research and public health
Implementers	Pragmatic training in management of research projects; discipline-specific education and training
Investigators	Education and training in clinical subspecialties (such as cardiology and infectious diseases), biomedical research, biostatistics, health services research, regulatory science, epidemiology, computational biology, genomics, and new technologies (such as imaging, cell and tissue engineering, and nanotechnology)
Academicians or Methodologists	Doctoral-level education in health research disciplines

[a] See Figure 3-1.
[b] Equipoise is the point at which a rational, informed person has no preference between two (or more) available treatments (Lilford and Jackson, 1995). In clinical research, the ethical concept of equipoise is satisfied when genuine uncertainty exists as to the comparative therapeutic benefits of the therapies in each arm of a clinical trial.
SOURCE: Bonham et al., 2012. *Developing a Robust Clinical Trials Workforce*. Discussion Paper, Institute of Medicine. (See Appendix E.)

Across the CTE workforce, increased demographic diversity—namely, greater levels of participation by racial and ethnic minorities—could help ensure that research conduct is relevant to, and research results serve the needs of, largely underserved communities. Those who experience health disparities often do not participate in trials at rates high enough to constitute subpopulations from which statistically significant findings are produced (e.g., Pollack, 2011). Inasmuch as current U.S. Census projections suggest that by 2020 nearly one in three Americans will be African American or Hispanic, improving the health of these populations is essential to maintaining and improving the health of the country as a whole. Similarly, higher rates of participation in clinical trials by people over age 65, and especially over age 85, could make trial results more relevant to the very large and expanding elderly population, given projections that 1 in 5 U.S. residents will be 65 or older by 2030 (Vincent and Velkoff, 2010). Clinical trials participation by overweight or obese people, people with chronic diseases, and residents of urban communities also will have to increase in order for research to be representative of the total population. Women and racial minorities remain underrepresented in the ranks of principal investigators. One study found that 16.9 percent of White physicians participate as principal investigators in clinical trials compared to 14 percent of African American physicians, 10.8 percent of Hispanic, and 9.6 percent of Asian physicians (Tufts Center for the Study of Drug Development, 2007). The study also found that 10.9 percent of female physicians participate as principal investigators compared to 16.9 percent of male physicians. The co-authors noted that, even if demographic parity is not achieved in all areas of the workforce, the CTE could benefit if researchers are skilled in engaging the community in clinical trials and able to accommodate demographic trends in designing, implementing, and analyzing clinical trials.

OPPORTUNITIES TO CREATE A SUSTAINABLE WORKFORCE FOR THE CLINICAL TRIALS ENTERPRISE

In a panel discussion, the session chair, panel presenters, Discussion Paper co-authors, and audience members reacted to and built upon the ideas contained in the Discussion Paper. Participants included session chair Sherine Gabriel, William J. and Charles H. Mayo Professor of Medicine and Epidemiology, Mayo Medical School; and panelists Briggs Morrison, Senior Vice President and Head of Worldwide Medical Excellence, Pfizer Inc.; and Rebecca Jackson, Associate Dean for Clinical Research, Professor of Medicine and Director of the Center for Women's Health at The Ohio State University. This section provides an integrated summary of their remarks and should not be construed as reflecting consensus or endorsement by the workshop participants, the planning committee, the Forum, or the National Academies.

The Public

The clinical trials "workforce" of the future may consist largely of patients themselves. Public participation in clinical trials could increase if biomedical knowledge is widely accepted as a "public good," benefiting everyone, so that people perceive a duty to contribute (Schaefer et al., 2009). Already, many patients and patient advocates, including disease-specific organizations, have exhibited a superior understanding of clinical trials. For example, the National Marfan Foundation says on its website that the organization "does not recommend switching from a beta blocker to losartan," pending results of a clinical trial of losartan still in progress (National Marfan Foundation, 2011). The National Foundation for Infantile Paralysis pioneered public support for clinical research in the early

20th century, partly through the March of Dimes, and this tradition continues with efforts such as the Love/Avon Army of Women, which enlists participants in breast cancer trials in collaboration with the American Association for Cancer Research and the National Breast Cancer Coalition. In the rare diseases clinical research network involving 93 diseases, patient advocacy groups participate in research through such activities as protocol development, study steering committee membership, and review of informed consent policies.

Formal credentialing of individuals also can facilitate broader public participation. In Cleveland, efforts are under way to provide certification in clinical research to community leaders, who then help develop specific research projects.

The low level of health literacy in the U.S. population is well documented (IOM, 2004, 2011c; Rudd et al., 2007). Teaching a basic medical vocabulary and the principles of clinical research in high schools could better prepare people to participate as volunteers in clinical trials, while also introducing more students, including minority students, to the possibility of careers in clinical research. Incorporating clinical research into the high school curriculum could lead to students' assisting their parents with participation in clinical research studies, including clinical trials. Several workshop participants noted that, given the pace of change in both medical science and health care delivery, the ability to be an "informed consumer" is essential to maintaining health and maximizing benefit from the health care system.

Community Practitioners

Negative physician attitudes toward research, often manifested through limited communication with patients about opportunities to participate in clinical trials, was mentioned by some participants as a major reason why clinical trials today struggle to recruit and retain patients. Only about 7 percent of adult Americans report that a physician has ever suggested to them that they participate in a clinical research study, although three-fourths say they would be very likely or somewhat likely to participate if asked (Research!America, 2007).

Physician behavior is a critical factor in applying research results to health care. Lauer noted that in the Occluded Artery Trial (OAT), no benefit was found to the common U.S. practice of using stents or balloon angioplasty to open occluded arteries that had not been opened within 12 hours following acute myocardial infarctions (AMIs) (Hochman et al., 2006). Clinical guidelines were revised in accordance with these findings, yet practices generally did not change in the several years immediately following release of the revised guidelines (Deyell et al., 2011). Moreover, according to Lauer, the study researchers experienced extraordinary difficulty recruiting U.S. physicians to take part in the study, and this recruitment difficulty is attributed largely to the fact that the study challenged the conventional wisdom about the benefits of opening persistently occluded arteries. Another workshop participant added that physician recruitment in OAT was further challenged by financial disincentives to the extent that a clinician's participation in the trial limited the number of artery–opening procedures she or he would be able to perform in compliance with the trial protocol. Another financial disincentive was that if the trial revealed the procedure to be unsafe or ineffective, physician caseloads and revenue would decrease.

According to some participants, the culture of research in North American medical schools appears to be diminishing. Part of physicians' reluctance to participate in, or apply findings from, clinical trials may stem from attitudes rooted in the Flexner reforms of medical education dating back a century ago, noted Califf. Under the Flexner model, the basis of medical practice is knowledge of human biology. Today it may make more sense for the basis of medical practice to consist of clinical evidence (albeit with an understanding of biology). Another partial explanation for inadequate attention to research in medical schools may be faculty members' relative lack of knowledge or comfort with research science.

According to Jackson, empiricism could be inculcated into undergraduate students, medical students, residents, and other future health professionals, such as dietitians, by teaching about the scientific investigations process and its relationship to health care, and by integrating clinical research into other coursework. In this way, students would learn to think of a working diagnosis as a hypothesis, and to view medical examinations and tests as an experiment to test the diagnostic hypothesis. It would be helpful for education to include use of research results and interpretation of statistical findings. It was suggested that, to introduce and take advantage of these changes, external pressures may be needed. Individual workshop participants highlighted several possible strategies for improving the education of community practitioners about research to help enhance their future participation in clinical trials:

- Revision of curricula in some medical schools, which may provide opportunities to introduce research problems into each educational module;
- Inclusion of questions about research in national medical board and nursing examinations; and
- Strengthening of medical school accreditation standards and requirements related to the teaching of research methods with the goal of increasing support for a culture of research.

An additional frontier of learning involves management of trials. Although some practitioners are very adept at managing logistics—a key skill in clinical research—others are not, and the teaching of management skills is not yet included in most health professions' educational curricula.

Implementers

Implementers are the people who conduct trials as a primary job function but are not engaged in the academic study of trial design methods. They (and others) will benefit from being taught to think in innovative ways and being trained to look at research problems from the perspective of patients and clinicians. It would be beneficial if education programs were refocused in order to meet not only gaps in knowledge but also gaps in methodology, implementation, and application, and to create cultural change. To this end, the NIH Clinical and Translational Science Awards (CTSAs) are striving to improve and increase training through a network of 60 medical research institutions. The program's training component includes a mentored clinical research scholar program at the postdoctoral level and tailored clinical research training for predoctoral students.

One core constituency of the implementers group is clinical research coordinators. Unfortunately, clinical research coordinators have been found to leave the field within 3 years, a waste of training and talent that apparently results from inadequate career paths. Indeed, retention of clinical research coordinators is now often considered a greater problem than attracting applicants to coordinator positions. Partly to promote the field and imbue it with the advantages of a recognized profession, efforts to develop an accreditation program for these professionals have begun at the University of Pennsylvania, and a Society of Clinical Research Associates has been created. With expertise in both management and clinical sciences, clinical research coordinators conceivably could be educated through master's degree programs jointly developed by medical and business schools.

Investigators

Investigators are the personnel charged with leading and designing clinical trials. This group would be composed of M.D.-, M.D./Ph.D.-, and Ph.D.-level investigators from a range of disciplines with the opportunity to supplement their expertise with specific training in translational and clinical research offered by the CTSAs. Paper co-authors suggested that the future transformation of AHSSs into IHSs will bridge translational gaps between discovery science and health care delivery and will require more of this highly trained cadre of clinical investigators.

Several workshop participants suggested that a sustainable and interesting career path is at least as important as, if not more important than, instituting formal training in the medical school curriculum. The rise of medical informatics may be instructive. Medical informatics is emerging as a board-certified specialty due to demand on the part of young physicians attracted to a field that hospitals and delivery systems find essential. Likewise, clinical research could become attractive if many more job positions were created.

In addition to bench researchers, it also is important to prepare people for positions in regulatory science,[2] notably within FDA. FDA regulations ensure the safety, efficacy, quality, and performance of products that represent about 25 cents of every dollar spent by American consumers. In the face of rapidly changing technology and increasingly complex products, FDA and other regulatory agencies must maintain their staff's scientific and technical expertise while responding as rapidly and effectively as possible to patients' needs and to public health emergencies.

A 2012 IOM report suggested the wide range of core competencies needed for professionals working in the regulatory sciences. In medicine, these competencies might include bioengineering, bioethics, clinical pharmacology, epidemiology, genetics, nutrition, public health, toxicology, and many others, going well beyond the disciplines traditionally associated with regulation, such as statistics and clinical research. In some cases, needed competencies may even be found outside the biomedical sciences in disciplines such as economics and sociology (IOM, 2012b).

Academicians and Methodologists

Academicians and methodologists are those who conduct research in new clinical trial methods and policies. This group of clinical investigators would consist of biostatisticians, epidemiologists, and health services researchers tasked with advancing and improving upon clinical trial methodologies. The workforce group would reside primarily in AHSSs, government, research institutes, and some larger industry groups that could provide protected time for research.

Investigators and academicians and methodologists are not entirely distinct from each other in that both design clinical trials. Ideally, these workforce groups will be taught to focus on what clinicians and patients need and will become proficient in behavioral skills and teamwork and even will become "design thinkers." According to several workshop

---

[2] FDA has defined regulatory science as the "science of developing new tools, standards, and approaches to assess the safety, efficacy, quality, and performance of FDA-regulated products" (FDA, 2010).

participants, the CTSA program and other initiatives have spurred the development of innovative research teams that tackle complex health and research challenges to identify ways to turn their discoveries into practical solutions to problems in patient care. Even at this high level, lifelong learning can help maintain and improve competencies, especially as scientists move from one career challenge to another in both private and public sectors.

SUSTAINING INSTITUTIONAL SUPPORT AND PATIENT ENGAGEMENT IN CLINICAL TRIALS

Clinical research gives the public hope. And you
cannot underestimate the power of that word.
—*John Gallin, NIH Clinical Center*

Models and Messages from the NIH Clinical Center[3]

An innovative and comprehensive approach to facilitating the conduct of clinical research has been developed by the NIH Clinical Center, a 240-bed facility located on the NIH campus in Bethesda, Maryland. The Clinical Center, which calls itself "America's Research Hospital," conducts a robust program of clinical research aimed at improving the treatment of both common and rare diseases and conditions. The approach was detailed in a keynote address by John Gallin, Director, NIH Clinical Center. Every patient at the Clinical Center is enrolled in a clinical study protocol and receives care free of charge (see Glossary in Appendix K for definition of protocol). The center's research portfolio consists mostly of Phase I and II investigations, rather than later-stage, confirmatory research. Studies are divided roughly in half between natural history studies of disease pathogenesis in patients with rare diseases and clinical trials.

NIH intramural clinical research benefits from the agency's adherences to seven "principles and processes" that it provides researchers: clinical informatics, data management, and protocol tracking; biostatistics support; quality assurance and quality improvement; protocol review; human resources and physical plant; training and education; and research participants, or research partners, as the term used at the Clinical Center. The Clinical Center has established systems to meet these needs for researchers, thereby substantially lightening investigators' administrative burdens (see Box 3-1). Some of the resources that NIH has developed to support its own intramural clinical trials program are increasingly being

---

[3] This section is based on the keynote address by John Gallin, Director, NIH Clinical Center.

BOX 3-1[a]
NIH Clinical Center Key Services for Researchers and Patients

- Services of protocol navigators, writers, and translators
- Office of Protocol Services support as a repository of NIH protocols that also prepares all reports to Congress and provides quality review of protocol actions, such as informed consent documents
- ProtoType, a web-based protocol writing tool that can be used, for example, in developing cost estimates and assessing regulatory compliance, and a "wizard" tool to help determine whether an investigator must submit an Investigational New Drug (IND) Application to FDA
- Biomedical Translational Information System, a web-based integrator of clinical and research data that offers investigators access to deidentified patient data, integrates data sources from multiple institutes, and provides an ontology for representation queries
- Assistance with recruitment and retention of study participants and with external communications, including media relations, use of social media, and outreach efforts, such as vaccine mobile clinics to facilitate vaccination studies
- Volunteer survey research on people's satisfaction with participation in studies; study participants are viewed as partners in clinical research
- Specialized services, including phenotyping, which is especially useful to researchers in rare diseases, as well as superior imaging services and pharmacy services that can formulate specialized products
- Training services, including NIH Curriculum on Clinical Research (introduction to the principles and practices of clinical research, principles of clinical pharmacology, and ethical and regulatory aspects of clinical research), an online course for clinical investigators on standards in clinical research, and a six-module clinical researcher sabbatical program lasting an average of three and a half months
- Community outreach activities, including a van that travels around the Washington metro area to make it easy for individuals who want to participate in a vaccine clinical trial to get examined and provide blood for purposes of the clinical trial
- Annual survey (focus group) of participants' perceptions of their research experiences. Aggregate survey data will identify best practices and drive improvements at the Clinical Center, and beyond (Kost et al., 2011)

---

[a] This box is based on the presentation by John Gallin, Director, NIH Clinical Center.

made available to external researchers. These resources are particularly useful for researchers who need more support than what their home institutions can offer. Making them more widely available also helps the Clinical Center fulfill its mandate to open its doors to extramural investigators.

Protocol navigators are a special feature of the Clinical Center's approach. Although their specific functions vary from one NIH Institute or Center to another, their role is to interface with components of NIH and to help overcome regulatory barriers. Figure 3-2 displays the National Institute of Allergy and Infectious Diseases (NIAID) navigators' functions. From 2009 to 2011, the Protocol Navigator Program at NIAID has conducted 29 initial protocol reviews, 10 protocol amendments, and 7 international studies serving 29 investigators from 10 different NIAID labs. The annual cost of the NIAID Protocol Navigator Program is $600,000 and staffs 1 navigation manager, 2 protocol navigators and 3 medical writers. To generate a larger pool of protocol navigators for intramural and extramural research support, the Clinical Center is developing a one-year training program intended as an alternative career path for research nurses, scientific writers, and IRB professionals to become versed in protocol navigation.

The Clinical Center's new vision statement reads: "The role of the NIH Clinical Center should be to serve as a state-of-the-art national resource, with resources optimally managed to enable both internal and external investigator use" (NIH, Scientific Management Review Board, 2010). The expansion from strictly intramural to joint intra- and extramural research activity is being introduced through a project to create partnerships between extramural and intramural researchers. A partnership program between basic scientists and clinical investigators also is being maintained, for the duration of current funding capacity.

Other Institutional Supports and Patient Engagement

This section is based on a panel discussion with John Gallin; Janet Tobias, CEO, Ikana Health; Annetine Gelijns, Co-chair, Department of Health Evidence and Policy, Mount Sinai School of Medicine; and Heather Snyder, Senior Associate Director for Scientific Grants, Alzheimer's Association International Research Grant Program. In the discussion, individual panelists and audience members identified challenges and opportunities to improve engagement in, and support of, clinical trials at the institutional and patient levels. This section provides an integrated summary of their remarks and discussions.

Public engagement is essential to the CTE but may constitute a weak link. Clinical trial recruitment and retention rates vary across disease area and provider, with AHSSs showing high variability.

Some barriers to participation by the public in clinical trials include

- lack of awareness of the benefits of engaging in clinical trials and the availability of relevant trials in which to participate (IOM, 2012a);

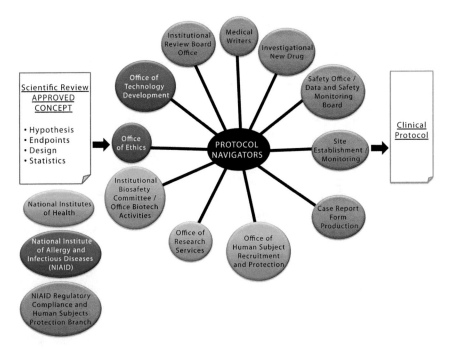

FIGURE 3-2 The protocol navigator interface at the National Institute of Allergy and Infectious Diseases (NIAID).
SOURCE: Gallin, J. 2011. Presentation at IOM workshop on Envisioning a Transformed Clinical Trials Enterprise in the United States: Establishing an Agenda for 2020. Figure created by H. Clifford Lane, NIAID, and publicly available.

- clinical trials designed without patient input and therefore lacking acceptability to the patients expected to participate in these studies;
- patient preferences for one treatment over another or the availability of a treatment outside the clinical trial setting;
- logistic hassles in participation (such as requirements of frequent patient visits, lab tests, and questionnaires); and
- inadequate reimbursement (for example, Medicare has paid for routine care in clinical trials since about 2000, but many private payers do not) which might lead to out-of-pocket expenses for trial participants.

Several strategies might be used to reduce these barriers. For example, Gelijns noted that a national coalition of patients, providers, and political leaders might promote change. On a more limited basis, an opportunity may exist to broaden the existing clinical trial networks that have been established by NIH to increase efficiency in research. These networks could include advocacy groups, community practitioners, and other stakeholders who could enrich trial design, logistics, recruitment, payment, and other aspects of studies. Networks might revolve around academic health and science center hubs and include community practitioners, whose patients could participate in trials through visits to their usual practitioner's office rather than to a distant research site. Engaging patients in the development of novel clinical trial designs and the determination of clinical end points may help in raising enrollment rates. Routine, effective communication with trial participants about study results also could improve people's sense of the value of the research effort. Collaboration between payers and the CTE, such as new FDA collaboration with CMS on innovative medical device use, could prove fruitful in ensuring both reimbursement and the application of research results to practice.

Clinical research gives people hope, noted John Gallin. To illustrate, parents enroll children in cancer studies at very high rates, as much as 90 percent. Advocacy groups have proved instrumental in promoting engagement in research on breast cancer, cystic fibrosis (CF), Alzheimer's disease, and other illnesses, especially when they have been viewed as impartial rather than favoring one treatment or trial over another. It might be useful to devote more resources to public engagement at earlier stages of research efforts, and to employ greater expertise in these communication efforts. Tobias noted that people are more willing to enroll in studies involving diseases perceived as life-threatening, such as cancer, and less willing to enroll in studies involving diseases, such as diabetes or Alzheimer's disease, that, even though they too are life-threatening and highly prevalent, are not perceived as such. A workshop participant also noted that beyond issues of disease severity, or perception of severity, a patient's interest in participating in a clinical trial is related to the availability of effective, acceptable treatments. A current trend in Alzheimer's disease research, according to Snyder, is to seek ways to identify patients as early as possible and to view the disease as a continuum.

There may be various education and communication strategies that could prove useful. Scientific education in elementary, middle, and high schools could enhance people's scientific literacy and improve physician–patient interactions. As mentioned in Chapter 2, the clinical trials workforce could also become skilled at incorporating the patient perspective into the design of clinical trials so as to make participation more attractive and acceptable to the public. Individually matching a patient with a clinical trial is another approach. When a 5-city survey found that a large proportion of primary care physicians were unaware of local trials and lacked time to find out about them, the Alzheimer's Association developed a program that has matched 3,300 patients with trials so far, said Snyder.

Enhancing public awareness might only be part of a larger remedy for improving participation in clinical research. In large part, recruitment is a matter of using the right language and communication techniques. To illustrate, mere education about clinical research and randomization may not suffice to increase recruitment rates, especially in the face of the heavy burden of participation. An evaluation of the "Get Randomised" media campaign in Scotland revealed that, although the campaign increased public awareness about clinical research, it did not increase the willingness of individuals to participate in clinical studies (Mackenzie et al., 2010).

4

Creating a New Business Model for Clinical Trials

Costs of clinical trials have been rising in the United States (DeVol et al., 2011). The workshop's third session, "Aligning Cultural and Financial Incentives," explored opportunities for developing a new business model for clinical trials based on the seamless integration of technological advances and research activities to realize increased efficiencies and reduced costs. Individual speakers also proposed greater harmonization of regulatory responsibilities and administrative processes. If such changes take place on a large scale, clinical trials could become more affordable and attractive to organizations, clinicians, and the public.

TRANSFORMING THE ECONOMICS OF CLINICAL TRIALS[1]

While the technology for gathering clinical data for research has evolved over time, the business model supporting this technology clearly has not evolved with each stage of technology transformation.
—*Judith Kramer, Duke University Medical Center; and Kevin Schulman, Duke University Medical Center*

---

[1] This section is based on the presentations and Discussion Paper by Judith Kramer, Associate Professor of Medicine, Duke University Medical Center, and Executive Director, Clinical Trials Transformation Initiative (CTTI), Duke Translational Medicine Institute; and Kevin Schulman, Professor of Medicine, Duke University Medical Center, and Gregory Mario and Jeremy Mario Professor of Business Administration, Fuqua School of Business. (See Appendix F for the Discussion Paper "Transforming the Economics of Clinical Trials.")

Advances in IT combined with business model transformation could combine to form a critical step in achieving transformation of the CTE through lower cost, faster, and better data quality of clinical trials according to a background paper prepared by Judith Kramer, Associate Professor of Medicine, Duke University Medical Center, and Executive Director, Clinical Trials Transformation Initiative (CTTI), Duke Translational Medicine Institute; and Kevin Schulman, Professor of Medicine, Duke University Medical Center, and Gregory and Jeremy Mario Professor of Business Administration, Fuqua School of Business. (See "Transforming the Economics of Clinical Trials" in Appendix F.) The entities involved in the conduct of clinical trials have not followed the cost-reduction trajectory of other technology-intensive industries and thus have not attained a business transformation sufficient to reap the economic benefits of technologic change. Instead, rapidly rising costs of U.S. clinical trials contribute to cost increases in developing innovative health products. For example, the estimated cost of developing one new drug has been suggested to range from $500 million to $2 billion (Adams and Brantner, 2006). The resulting high cost of conducting clinical trials constricts the pipeline for new drug development, limits the accretion of knowledge about drugs that are produced, deters a focus on innovation and improvements in trial design and conduct, and impedes the investigation of important public health inquiries.

Increasing costs stem in part from obstacles that exist within regulatory pathways or stem from administrative inefficiencies, including increasingly complex clinical trial protocols, abundant requirements issued by various levels of government and different governments and not harmonized to ensure consistency, and excessively risk-averse interpretations of regulations by trial sponsors. An example of the last is 100 percent source documentation of all clinical trial data even though regulators—both FDA and the European Medicines Agency (EMA)—do not require it. Some new structures, such as CROs, have arisen to help trial sponsors operate in the complex research environment. CROs are focused on efficiently conducting clinical trials according to current standards and client expectations and do not have as their mandate a goal of advancing innovation in clinical trial design and performance. According to some observers, CROs may improve efficiency for trial sponsors, but their business practices may also contribute to the current cost structure of clinical research.

According to the authors, new information technologies conceivably could alter the conduct of clinical trials. For instance, electronic data capture (EDC)—using a computerized system to gather clinical data in a clinical trial—has the potential to reduce total costs, prevent errors, and conserve the time expended by physicians, nurses, and data coordinators by replacing multiple paper entries on patients' clinical progress with onsite, electronic entry. EHRs could also reduce recruitment and site-screening costs and, furthermore, could enable direct-to-patient research, limiting the involvement of physician intermediaries. Pfizer recently initiated the nation's first clinical trial, in support of an IND application, that recruits participants over the Internet (Mansell, 2011). Smart phones are another technology that can improve communication within research programs and facilitate recruitment of participants in trials. However, research entities continue to rely on legacy systems, such as freestanding site-specific monitoring mechanisms and IRBs, rather than having these functions centralized among all or most sites involved in the same trial. So long as research organizations persist in overlaying the old business model atop the new technologies, many potential efficiencies will not be realized.

A broad approach to ensure the business model for clinical trials keeps pace with technology and information needs and capabilities could be based on a research agenda that examines how research is conducted today. This research would point the way forward in terms of identifying potential issues, and pathways, to reach business transformation of clinical trials. The research agenda would be reassessed every 2 to 5 years to ensure that business and regulatory mechanisms keep pace with technologic advances and other changes in the economic, scientific, and health care environment surrounding the CTE. Suggested pathways and opportunities for moving research business models forward would therefore reflect findings that emanate from a forward-looking research agenda that considers the seamless integration of technology into research. Also, harmonization of regulations among multiple agencies, including different levels of government in the United States and different countries (including the European Union), could reduce the cost of monitoring trials. Regulatory relief also could come in the form of the establishment of safe harbors for business process innovation—to allow sponsors to follow certain promising pathways before regulations have been developed and finalized. Furthermore, enhanced clinical research education of health professionals could equip practitioners to contribute to strategic efforts to develop new ways to streamline clinical trials into clinical practice. Organizations that play a role in clinical research could reorient themselves toward economic efficiency, shed "sunk costs" such as legacy systems that no longer are needed, avoid overly cumbersome mechanisms for applying regulatory controls, and embrace new information technologies. Possible strategies mentioned during the presentation of the Discussion Paper and discussion with the workshop audience for resolving economic inefficiencies in clinical trials are summarized in Box 4-1.

Feasible new business models could emerge to replace the highly labor-intensive and regulation-laden clinical trials system that predomi-

---

BOX 4-1[a]
Selected Potential Strategies for Avoiding Unnecessary Costs in Clinical Trials

The following actions suggested by Kramer and Schulman and individual workshop participants could facilitate the creation of new business models for clinical research that integrate technologic advances:

- Develop a national research agenda, based partly on "research-on-research" findings, to guide business transformation based on the next generation of technology;
- Harmonize regulations issued by different agencies and governments;
- Move away from excessively risk-averse interpretations of regulations by research organizations;
- Enhance clinical research education of health professionals, so they can help design more efficient and meaningful research programs;
- Apply new information technologies, such as web-based clinical trials and smart phones, in place of outmoded mechanisms;
- Use EDC and EHRs to apply clinical data to research, replacing paper-based legacy systems;
- Reconsider costly regulatory controls, such as the Health Insurance Portability and Accountability Act (HIPAA) regulations applied to clinical research, and provide safe harbors for business process innovation;
- Engage in more strategic planning and consider new organizational structures for entities conducting clinical trials; and
- Focus compliance monitoring and other oversight on areas of greatest risk, and introduce expedited review and flexibility as appropriate.

---

[a] The information in this box is based on the presentations of Kramer and Schulman (2011) and Discussion Paper by Judith Kramer, Associate Professor of Medicine, Duke University Medical Center, and Executive Director, CTTI, Duke Translational Medicine Institute; and Kevin Schulman, Professor of Medicine, Duke University Medical Center, and Gregory Mario and Jeremy Mario Professor of Business Administration, Fuqua School of Business (see Appendix F for the Discussion Paper "Transforming the Economics of Clinical Trials"); and discussions with the workshop audience.

---

nates today. The adoption of new business models could be facilitated by the engagement of all sectors in the conceptualization of business transformation.[2] The uptake of new clinical trial business models could increase return on investment and introduce greater predictability and efficiency as a consistent attribute of the CTE.

---

[2] For example, currently, the CTTI, a collaboration between Duke University and FDA, is undertaking to combine the perspectives of more than 50 stakeholder organizations to develop new approaches and begin to point the way toward a new model for clinical trials.

IDENTIFYING OPPORTUNITIES TO IMPROVE
REGULATORY FRAMEWORKS FOR CLINICAL TRIALS[3]

Regulations are sometimes an excuse and
sometimes a huge, real issue.
—Kevin Schulman, Duke University Medical Center

Regulatory Harmonization

Paul Eisenberg, Senior Vice President, Global Regulatory Affairs and Safety, Amgen Inc., discussed regulatory challenges from an industry perspective, focusing on the need for greater regulatory harmonization (see also Chapter 5). According to Eisenberg, FDA's IND application process in the United States, while not particularly onerous in any single respect, is overall more cumbersome than corresponding European or other foreign processes. A selection of problematic processes associated with U.S. regulatory frameworks suggested by Eisenberg includes

- the use of form 1572 (which other nations actually discourage) for clinical investigators;
- thorough and time-consuming FDA review of the formulation and processes that led to the development of the clinical trial materials used in a study under the IND process. By contrast, in Europe, products developed in accordance with Good Manufacturing Practice (GMP) guidelines are deemed safe, and trial practices that meet Good Clinical Practice (GCP) principles are deemed acceptable. In some countries, a clinical trial can begin with a "clinical trial notification," or a single IRB approval of the trial protocol;
- undeveloped regulatory framework for the co-development of devices and drugs under the IND process in the United States. In the past decade, an increasing number of pharmaceutical products in development have come from large molecules that, by nature, are more complex in their delivery mechanisms to patients. Thus, large-molecule products in development might require syringes or other devices to be developed simultaneously so that individuals can benefit from these novel therapeutics;
- the evolving and somewhat confusing mechanism for reporting adverse events experienced by clinical trial participants (including immediate reporting of "serious" and unexpected events experienced by participants);

---

[3] This section is based on remarks made by Paul Eisenberg, Senior Vice President, Global Regulatory Affairs and Safety, Amgen Inc., and the Discussion Paper "Developing a Clinical Trials Infrastructure" (see Appendix G).

- management of privacy protections under the HIPAA privacy regulations; and
- frequent, time-consuming inspections conducted by multiple regulatory authorities at research sites outside the United States.

The United States is not always a regulatory minefield. For example, ethical review—the IRB process—actually tends to be more efficient in the United States than in other countries. Nevertheless, as a consequence of existing regulation-related challenges, Eisenberg said, pharmaceutical research and manufacturing firms that would otherwise prefer to conduct clinical trials at U.S. academic health and science centers may find themselves drawn instead to foreign venues for research.

Given the fact that research is conducted in many countries, opportunities for substantial collaboration and regulatory harmonization exist. One is the potential for a standard international nomenclature—to describe drug reactions, for example. Another opportunity that could be explored is the establishment of a worldwide clinical trial database, similar to ClinicalTrials.gov, but with broader participation from around the world. Joint or coordinated inspections for GCP constitute a third potential opportunity for international harmonization.

OPPORTUNITIES FOR ALIGNING CULTURAL AND FINANCIAL INCENTIVES IN CLINICAL TRIALS

In a panel discussion, the session chair, panel presenters, Discussion Paper co-authors, and audience members reacted to and built upon the ideas contained in the Discussion Paper. Participants included session chair, Arthur Rubenstein, Professor of Medicine, Division of Endocrinology, Raymond and Ruth Perelman School of Medicine, University of Pennsylvania; Richard Rudick, Professor of Medicine and Hazel Prior Hostetler Chair of Neurology, Cleveland Clinic Lerner College of Medicine of Case Western Reserve University; Christopher Beardmore, CEO, Translational Research Management; and Scott Steele, Director of Research Alliances, University of Rochester. This section provides an integrated summary of their remarks and should not be construed as reflecting consensus or endorsement by the workshop participants, the planning committee, the Forum, or the National Academies.

The health care system is adopting widespread transformative practices, such as moving toward employment of physicians by large health care delivery systems (as opposed to individual physicians in private practice), use of performance measures in determining reimbursement, distance health monitoring, and other major changes. But, according to several participants, transformation of the CTE and of the health care system are proceeding on different tracks, even within institutions, such as AHSSs.

Cultural and Other Barriers

Workshop participants mentioned several possible cultural, economic, and regulatory barriers impeding transformation of the CTE into new business models. It was suggested by one workshop participant that older researchers are often less comfortable with new information technologies than younger researchers, which might hinder their involvement in the latest clinical trials. Another barrier is that regulatory and legal concerns make some people fearful of attempting innovations that could create liability problems for their institution. Some workshop participants noted that the public is not highly informed about science and research, and that there may be a casual attitude that is shared by political leaders and even clinical practitioners. In the current health care system, academic medicine is largely separate from community practice, and community practitioners may not view their job function as involving research. Rudick noted that clinical research and clinical investigators cannot function, let alone thrive, when they operate separately from the health care system. He stressed the need to integrate clinical trials, and more broadly clinical research, into the U.S. health care system in order to realize a truly transformed CTE.

It was noted that although the pluralistic U.S. health care system has several advantages over a monolithic system, such as avoiding some wasteful expenditures for large systems before they are piloted on a small scale, the fragmentation makes it difficult to achieve change quickly and universally. Cultural change also could be spurred by new regulatory approaches. For example, it was noted that establishment of an opt-out mechanism, where people are presumed to approve use of their patient records for research purposes unless they specify otherwise, could facilitate the secondary use of patient data for research purposes and promote the expectation of public participation in research.

Reimbursement and Economic Incentives

It is of signal importance for third-party payers to cover the costs of participation in clinical trials. Patients in trials can incur costs greater than patients in routine health care. Also, rational budgeting of clinical trials by sponsors is impossible without knowing which expenses are research administrative costs, to be paid by sponsors, and which are routine care costs, which may be required to be paid by insurers or patients. Some states already require payers to cover the routine medical care costs of patient participation in clinical trials. Section 10103(c) of the Patient Protection and Affordable Care Act requires coverage of routine patient care costs associated with clinical trials, with no discrimination against clinical trial participants, by the beginning of 2014.

An additional dimension of the reimbursement landscape is the fragmented nature of the U.S. health care system, including the existence of many payers. This fragmentation makes it difficult both to clarify which payer is responsible for covering the costs of a clinical trial and to have consistent and universal transformation of the business models for clinical trials. However, one participant noted that, because each payer makes its own coverage and payment decisions, an opportunity exists for providers to develop an innovative payment approach through negotiation with an individual payer (akin to a payer-specific demonstration program). Beardmore noted the feeling of some community oncologists that they are marginalized in discussions of cancer care policy and reimbursement reform despite the expectation that they will enthusiastically support and implement the programs and policies being developed (Kolodziej, 2011).

He also noted that with respect to reimbursement, many large payers are moving toward value-based insurance design, in which payers link reimbursement levels to evidence on health outcomes to reduce waste (IOM, 2007; Kapowich, 2010). One workshop participant suggested that this move indicates that cultural change about the value of research and evidence could ideally be partnered with a change in payment systems to demand (or "pull," as opposed to "push") more knowledge about treatments.

In addition to adequate compensation for patients and healthy volunteers participating in research, Eisenberg noted that insufficient compensation for clinical investigators is a problem that contributes to low levels of participation in and leadership of trials in the United States. Rudick also noted that there currently is no effective financing mechanism in place for clinical investigators in academic medicine, resulting in an unstable and unattractive career path.

Informatics

EDC, directed by a neutral entity operating via a system of cloud computing, can connect individual systems used by health care systems and research organizations. This interoperable approach could obviate the need for one unified data system. Alternatively, a central data repository could be established, with universally retrievable information about the capacity of research sites, the credentials of investigators, protection of human subjects, training, and other topics, thereby eliminating the need for the laborious and wasteful gathering of information to support each new trial.

Many informatics products now are legacy-driven. An AHSS that has invested in separate systems for billing and research does not have incentives to replace both systems with a new, integrated product. Different academic institutions have their own systems, and little interoperability exists. While federal regulators, health care providers, and the IT industry focus primarily on the "meaningful use"[4] of EHRs, according to a workshop participant they are not sufficiently investing in connectivity and the use of EHRs in the health care setting for clinical trials. Consequently, the records of patients who receive care from different providers, health systems, or academic institutions are all incomplete. It was suggested by one workshop participant to start increasing efficiency and interoperability by merging information for compliance systems such as financial disclosure forms. Billing, scheduling, and other processes also could be combined.

International Competition

Many participants noted that the United States will have to invest more heavily to remain competitive in the field of clinical research and to achieve more effective and value-driven health care. While other countries are increasing their commitment to medical research, in recent decades U.S. health policy concerns have been concentrated on cost containment. Clinical research has not been central to the discussion, even though research could lead to a significant reduction in expenditures for medically unnecessary procedures, which contribute to an estimated $750 billion to $765 billion of excess in annual U.S. health expenditures (IOM, 2010b).

Workshop participants expressed differing views about the best way to meet the challenge of globalization in clinical trials. One view was that it may make sense to let other countries undertake industry-driven studies, of the type regulated by FDA, while the United States moves into quality improvement and clinical effectiveness research as an area of growth. A contrasting view was that, to the extent clinical trials are moving offshore due to excessive U.S. research costs, this is a loss to the United States. In this view, research should be conducted in the United States if the results are to be applied to U.S. populations specifically. Another

---

[4] The HITECH Act, part of the American Recovery and Reinvestment Act of 2009, allowed CMS to provide financial incentives to health providers for the adoption and "meaningful use" of certified EHR technology. Meaningful use entails three components: (1) the use of certified EHR technology in a meaningful manner, such as e-prescribing; (2) the use of certified EHR technology for electronic exchange of health information to improve quality of health care; and (3) the use of certified EHR technology to submit clinical quality and other measures. For more information, visit https://www.cms.gov/EHRIncentivePrograms/30_Meaningful_Use.asp (accessed March 28, 2012).

type of viewpoint offered at the workshop identified spillover benefits to conducting clinical trials in the United States. Trials are educational opportunities because knowledge of, or participation in, clinical trials facilitates dialogue among clinicians about developing medical evidence for new treatments or comparing products or interventions already in use. Clinical trials are also a source of jobs. And finally, clinical trials can result in improved clinical care for trial participants.

Building Consortia to Create Conditions for Change

When the U.S. semiconductor industry faced strong pressure from Japanese competition and other forces, a Semiconductor Manufacturing Technology consortium (SEMATECH) was formed to create elements of a single manufacturing infrastructure, supported with the pooling of funds and public–private partnerships. The consortium concept may be applicable to the challenges facing the CTE, according to Steele. The creation of consortia could enhance the current clinical trials infrastructure. Already the Biomarkers Consortium, managed by the Foundation for the NIH (FNIH), is developing common adaptive trial designs. The CTSAs and academic medical centers share training programs, improve common understanding about regulatory requirements, improve informatics, develop model clinical trial agreements, and achieve other infrastructure enhancements across the CTSA institutions. The consortia model also could help overcome cultural barriers to CTE transformation, by resolving problems in leadership and governance. For example, Steele suggested that a consortium could be developed to revamp the weighty IRB structure as currently used in clinical research. Interagency coordination also can be improved through coordinating councils with multiagency input.

5

Building an Infrastructure to Support Clinical Trials

As noted in previous chapters, the existing clinical trials infrastructure[1] is considered by many participants in Forum activities to be inadequate to meet the requirements of a transformed CTE that would promote the efficient development of new and effective treatments, develop valid and reliable evidence about the clinical effectiveness of health care treatments, undergird a learning health system, and gain the confidence and widespread engagement of the public, health care providers, and policy makers. The clinical trials infrastructure is currently developed on a trial-by-trial basis, or in a sponsor-specific manner, resulting in "one-off" trials that bring together substantial resources that are subsequently disbanded. In previous and ongoing Forum discussions, many participants in Forum activities have suggested that efforts to develop a consistent and reliable clinical trials infrastructure that lived beyond the single trial could increase the efficiency and effectiveness of the entire CTE.

Individual workshop participants described major infrastructure deficits and practical ideas for shoring it up and converting weaknesses into strengths. The discussion echoed a number of comments made in previous sessions and centered on current challenges and directions for solutions in the areas of data gathering and processing, investigator train-

---

[1] The clinical trials infrastructure refers to the necessary resources (human capital, financial support, patient participants, information systems, regulatory pathways, and institutional commitment) and the manner in which they are organized and brought together to conduct a clinical trial.

53

ing, patient and practitioner engagement, institutional resources, and the coordination and organization of clinical trial resources.

GAPS AND CHALLENGES IN THE CURRENT CLINICAL TRIALS INFRASTRUCTURE[2]

A key objective of health care reform in the United States is to encourage use of the most effective therapies and implementation strategies. This will require multiple types of clinical trials in many different settings.
—*Paul Eisenberg, Amgen Inc.; Petra Kaufmann, National Institute of Neurological Disorders and Stroke (NINDS); Ellen Sigal, Friends of Cancer Research; and Janet Woodcock, Center for Drug Evaluation and Research, FDA*

Clinical trials in the United States have become too expensive, difficult to enroll, inefficient to implement, and ineffective to support the development of new medical products, or the clinical effectiveness of these products, under modern scientific standards of evidence. This critique is expressed in the Discussion Paper prepared by Paul Eisenberg, Amgen Inc.; Petra Kaufmann, Director, Office of Clinical Research, National Institute of Neurological Disorders and Stroke (NINDS), NIH; Ellen Sigal, Chair and Founder, Friends of Cancer Research; and Janet Woodcock, Director, Center for Drug Evaluation and Research, FDA. (See "Developing a Clinical Trials Infrastructure" in Appendix G). Ultimately, the purpose of CTE transformation is to facilitate development of more efficient and effective drugs and treatments, partly through continuous improvement of health care. A broad-based, sustainable infrastructure could support multiple types of clinical trials in different settings. Box 5-1 shows some of the elements of the clinical trials infrastructure that could be transformed.

A leading shortcoming of today's CTE is low participation rates by patients and the public. To increase participation, the paper suggests the creation of clinical trial networks that are one of the following: disease-specific; created through CTSAs for a constellation of diseases or oriented around a specific subpopulation (e.g., children); or a "hub-and-spoke" arrangement between AHSSs and community health care providers. The success of CF advocates illustrates the power of a network to initiate and

---

[2] This section is based on the presentations and Discussion Paper by Paul Eisenberg, Senior Vice President, Global Regulatory Affairs and Safety, Amgen Inc.; Petra Kaufmann, Director, Office of Clinical Research, National Institute of Neurological Disorders and Stroke (NINDS), NIH; Ellen Sigal, Chair and Founder, Friends of Cancer Research (unable to attend workshop); and Janet Woodcock, Director, Center for Drug Evaluation and Research, FDA. (See Appendix G for the Discussion Paper "Developing a Clinical Trials Infrastructure.")

BOX 5-1[a]
Elements of the Clinical Trials Infrastructure
Discussed at the Workshop

- Investigator recruitment
- Regulatory approval to conduct a clinical trial (e.g., IND in the United States)
- Contractual agreements between sponsors, institutions, and investigators
- Participant recruitment plan
- Coordination of global investigators and research sites
- Quality control systems
- Data collection, management, and analysis
- Data standards
- Communication of results
- Registration of trials and results with ClinicalTrials.gov

---

[a] This box is based on the Discussion Paper by Paul Eisenberg, Senior Vice President, Global Regulatory Affairs and Safety, Amgen Inc.; Petra Kaufmann, Director, Office of Clinical Research, NINDS, NIH; Ellen Sigal, Chair and Founder, Friends of Cancer Research (unable to attend workshop); and Janet Woodcock, Director, Center for Drug Evaluation and Research, FDA. (See Appendix G for the Discussion Paper "Developing a Clinical Trials Infrastructure.")

---

implement clinical trials, as this advocacy community has been highly influential in promoting extensive research on the disease. Several organizations in the United States and United Kingdom jointly funded a recently reported study (Ramsey et al., 2011). Woodcock pointed to this study as an example of how a network of organizations can collaborate to sponsor studies that contribute to medical knowledge. In the study, at least five organizations—a pharmaceutical manufacturer, the Cystic Fibrosis Foundation Therapeutic Development Center, NIH, and two British entities—funded a multisite RCT of a drug that increases the effectiveness of the CF transmembrane conductance regulator protein; the study found substantial improvements in weeks 2 through 48 (Ramsey et al., 2011). This type of effort, Woodcock noted, integrates research and clinical care and leads to continuous quality improvement through rigorous evaluation of interventions.[3]

---

[3] Since the workshop, FDA approved a new therapy, Kalydeco, in January 2012 to treat CF patients with a specific genetic mutation (approximately 4 percent of CF patients, or 1,200 individuals, have the mutation targeted by this new drug). The new drug is the first personalized treatment that targets a specific abnormal protein product of a specific gene in a subset of CF patients. The Cystic Fibrosis Foundation partnered with drug developer Vertex Pharmaceuticals to develop and study the drug in the relevant CF patient population. The partnership that led to the approval of this new therapy could provide a model

Robert Califf, Duke University Medical Center, noted that, as research networks grow and expand, it will be important to prevent them from becoming ossified or complicating opportunities to collaborate with external researchers.

Web-based innovations also could meet other infrastructure gaps. A participant noted that the infrastructure of the future could consist of web-based trials now being piloted, with a single "virtual" investigator and trial participants nationwide.

Some relief from the need to comply with many different requirements of multiple federal agencies has come from the Common Rule, or Federal Policy for the Protection of Human Subjects, originally adopted in 1991 and amended in 2005.[4] This regulation, with extensive new updates now under consideration, in effect harmonizes the approaches of some 17 federal agencies on IRB-related matters (HHS, 2011). Issues currently under consideration in review of the Common Rule include mandating a central IRB for multisite domestic studies; informed consent for future use of bio-specimens for research purposes (along with harmonization of Common Rule and HIPAA requirements on this subject); and requiring that even relatively small organizations provide extensive data security safeguards (CenterWatch, 2011; HHS, 2011). Additional relief from regulatory challenges could come through the auspices of the International Conference on Harmonisation of Technical Requirements for Registration of Pharmaceuticals for Human Use, a forum for the industry and regulatory authorities in the United States, Europe, and Japan to rationalize international regulations.

ESTABLISHING AN INFRASTRUCTURE TO SUPPORT A TRANSFORMED CLINICAL TRIALS ENTERPRISE

I am concerned that the message is coming through that clinical trials are all good, more clinical trials are better, and we need to make it easier to do more. . . . [G]ood clinical trials are good, bad clinical trials are not good.
—Deborah Zarin, ClinicalTrials.gov, National Library of Medicine

---

for future drug development and patient group collaborations. For more information visit http://www.fda.gov/NewsEvents/Newsroom/PressAnnouncements/ucm289633.htm (accessed March 28, 2012) and http://blogs.fda.gov/fdavoice/index.php/2012/01/how-science-and-strategic-collaboration-led-to-a-new-personalized-cystic-fibrosis-treatment-for-some-patients/ (accessed March 28, 2012).

[4] The Common Rule is based on HHS' basic regulation on Protection of Human Subjects (45 CFR 46, subpart A). Amendments were proposed in 76 (143) *Federal Register* (FR) 44512-44531 (July 26, 2011), comment period extended 76 (170) FR 54408 (September 1, 2011).

Responding to the Discussion Paper were Louis Fiore, Director, VA Cooperative Studies Program Coordinating Center, VA Boston Healthcare System; Michael King Jolly, Senior Vice President, Quintiles Drug Development Innovation; and Karen Margolis, Director of Clinical Research, HealthPartners Research Foundation, during a panel session moderated by Clyde Yancy, Northwestern University. Yancy noted that clinical practice guidelines—and even approvals of medical devices or other modalities—often lack a firm evidence base. Some panels responsible for clinical practice guidelines rely on data from other countries with a different population mix or clinical approach, data from a limited population (such as men only), or the results of trials for which the clinical end points were not developed in conjunction with patients. In short, too often there is no rational business model for developing evidence to support clinical guidelines, utilizing the dedicated services of a stable cadre of researchers within a single institution. Fiore, Jolly, and Margolis described the evolving and promising research capacity, built around large patient populations, of the VA, PACeR, and HMO (health maintenance organization) Research Network (HMORN), respectively. Disruptive ideas include

- *a patient-centric approach,* as opposed to the current approach that includes a selection bias in recruiting patients for a trial, as participants often are recruited only when they present to a particular provider;
- *a hospital approach,* with new strategies, similar to reduced payment for avoidable readmissions, which have served as a powerful incentive for change; and
- *incentives and centralized training for investigators,* combined with an end to the stigma associated with conducting industry-sponsored research.

Clinical Research Infrastructure at the VA[5]

Fiore discussed clinical research in the VA. More than 100 VA centers are approved for research, and staff is allocated time for the effort to conduct it. Every VA hospital has a research office and a nonprofit subsidiary to handle financial transactions. Because VA hospitals, and not a separate academic institution, are the grantees, the VA hospitals can collect indirect costs under the grants, thus providing greater incentives and support for research within the VA. The extensive VA research infrastructure includes the Office of Research and Development with, among other features, a

---

[5] This section is based on the presentation by Louis Fiore, Director, VA Cooperative Studies Program Coordinating Center, VA Boston Healthcare System.

centralized IRB; monitoring, pharmacy, and training facilities; and the ability to conduct small observational pilot studies to assist the development of larger research projects. The Genomic Informatics System for Integrative Science (GenISIS), perhaps the VA research "crown jewel," is an IT environment that uses both phenotypic and biologic data to facilitate the recruitment, enrollment, and analysis of people in clinical trials, especially studies involving genomic medicine. GenISIS provides numerous applications and databases, performance computing and data storage, and links to external data sources as well as patient records. Other VA advantages in conducting research include a large and stable patient population; a model EHR system, coupled with secondary use of data to identify patients meeting particular research criteria; and a secure clinical data warehouse (VA Informatics and Computing Infrastructure, or VINCI). Emerging VA programs include point-of-care research (using EHRs for randomization and workflow analysis) and development of the Million Veterans Program genomic research preconsented population, which will include banked biologic specimens as well as other resources. Also under development is the use of EHRs to identify patients who meet criteria for individual studies; this outreach activity will complement the patient portal where veterans can learn about, and enroll in, studies. Finally, expanding VA research resources to include DoD personnel will make the system even more powerful.

Partnership to Advance Clinical Electronic Research[6]

Jolly described PACeR, a consortium of 13 hospitals in New York State and many other inpatient and ambulatory care providers (see also Chapter 2) using an open-source platform for research. Established in 2010, PACeR is a public–private partnership intended to develop economically sustainable businesses to support translational medical research across the nation. Figure 5-1 depicts PACeR's capacity to standardize clinical research and complete clinical databases.

PACeR is both an operating system and a series of applications, using cloud computing technologies. Oracle is a partner and is involved in building greater interoperability into the system. Consistent with Fiore's comments regarding the VA, infrastructure capacity is key to PACeR, and standards—affecting policies, practice guidelines, procedures, methods, technologies, and data—are the key to interoperability. With respect to data, common standards dictionaries are used, so data from institutions with different data systems, or different versions of the same system, can be matched.

---

[6] This section is based on the presentation by Michael King Jolly, Senior Vice President, Quintiles Drug Development Innovation.

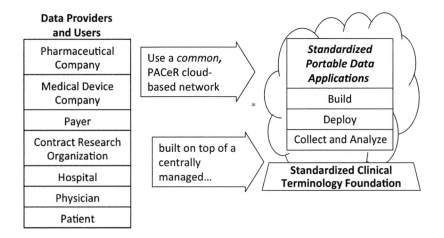

FIGURE 5-1 The PACeR (Partnership to Advance Clinical electronic Research) system fills the EMR clinical data gaps and captures uniform data across all clinical data capture sites, which is needed for evidence-based research.
SOURCE: Jolly, 2011. Presentation at IOM workshop on Envisioning a Transformed Clinical Trials Enterprise in the United States: Establishing an Agenda for 2020.

PACeR brings providers of information and buyers of information into a common space. It can generate new information through queries, and each institution can access the full array of data. In addition, PACeR provides patients with a portal, called MediGuard, for learning about studies for which they may meet eligibility criteria.

HMO Research Network[7]

Margolis described HMORN, a consortium of 19 large integrated health service providers serving people of all ages and other characteristics in all major regions of the country. Because HMORN includes several disease networks—on vaccine safety, cancer, cardiovascular diseases, mental health, and other areas—it is, in a sense, a network of networks, able to facilitate longitudinal studies. It functions as a virtual data warehouse, with data residing at each site but accessible to all members and thus capable of being consolidated. Each site has staff with sub-

---

[7] This section is based on the presentation by Karen Margolis, Director of Clinical Research, HealthPartners Research Foundation.

stantial programming and informatics expertise. Data are derived from tumor registries, mortality records, pharmacy orders, and, under development, even dental records. Costs of care can be calculated easily. To date, HMORN activity has concentrated on observational studies, but clinical studies and pragmatic trials are anticipated. Facilities include a voluntary central IRB and streamlined contracting. In addition, HMOs serve as a natural vehicle for contacting practitioners and for disseminating and using research findings.

During the discussion following panelist presentations, Marissa Miller, NHLBI, NIH, noted the success of the Interagency Registry for Mechanically Assisted Circulatory Support (INTERMACS), a national registry for patients who are receiving mechanical circulatory support device therapy to treat advanced heart failure. Miller highlighted that the NHLBI-funded registry was created with buy-in from stakeholders across the clinical research enterprise—CMS, FDA, academia, industry, scientists, and clinicians—who together developed rigorous data definitions, extensive data collection, and auditing processes for the registry. Use of the patient data in this robust registry has resulted in multiple research publications advancing medical evidence and guiding improvements in technology as devices to treat advanced heart failure evolve. Recently, the registry data has also been used in conducting clinical trials. INTERMACS serves a dual function: it (1) develops common definitions and a reporting system for adverse events and (2) generates a reference population for clinical trials, effectively streamlining the startup of clinical trials by removing the necessity to recruit a control population.

Table 5-1 provides an integrated summary of some the infrastructure challenges and possible directions for transformation cited in the Discussion Paper and presentations by Eisenberg, Kaufmann, and Woodcock and noted by individual workshop participants and audience members.

TABLE 5-1 Some Clinical Trials Infrastructure Challenges and Possible Courses of Action Mentioned at the Workshop

Challenge	Possible Course of Action
Insufficient evidence to support real-world clinical practice	• Multiple trials, in various settings, to generate more complete results that are relevant to clinical practice; • Increased input from practitioners and patients into development of trials; • Post clinical questions online; • IHSs' creation of a disease problem list to guide improvements in identifying study topics and designing trials or choosing the appropriate research method to answer the question being posed; and • Greater involvement of payers, employers, health system CEOs, and others in developing research tools and clinical trials to produce more relevant findings (e.g., building from the success of INTERMACS discussed above).
Insufficient engagement and participation in clinical trials by community health care providers and the public	• Design clinical trials that are appropriate and attractive from a patient's perspective—consider outcomes meaningful to the patient population and society; • Recruit participants through online networks; • Provide patients with standardized information on clinical trials, and develop a participation card similar to organ donation cards; • Web-based clinical trials that facilitate participation nationwide; • Alert clinicians when a patient meets criteria for participation in a trial, using EHRs and clinical trial identifiers; and • Increased encouragement and advocacy of participation in research by professional medical societies.
Lack of coordination—trials are conducted in a one-off manner	• Online trial infrastructure created through public–private partnerships; • Greater use of research coordinators; • Implement national research labs (similar to those supported by the Department of Energy) with core budgeting and a more engineered system of health learning; • Standardized online training programs and credentialing of investigators; and • Access to investigator track records (e.g., success recruiting patients to participate in clinical trials to date, ability to submit timely clinical trial data to coordinating centers) by research centers conducting clinical trials.

continued

TABLE 5-1 Continued

Challenge	Possible Course of Action
Poor communication about trials	• Develop opportunities for meaningful communication among patients, researchers, and community physicians about clinical trials; • Provide more information online about trials, perhaps through a user-friendly interface to ClinicalTrials.gov; • Transparent and reliable communication of trial results to the public through a patient portal; and • Facilitate remote clinical trial participation through mobile and web-based technologies so that patients do not need to visit research centers or physician offices for recording of progress.
Regulatory and administrative barriers	• Standardized contracts to reduce trial start-up delays; • Online protocol tools and common technical documents for applications to conduct trials; • Harmonize international requirements for reporting adverse events; • Creation of a universal numerical scheme to identify clinical trials across the world; • Build the U.S. regulatory framework for co-development of new drugs and the devices to administer them; • Harmonize clinical research site inspections; • Centralized IRBs, and other forms of relief under HHS Common Rule (see text below); and • More flexible FDA and NIH processes for determining type of trial appropriate for a drug investigation phase or research question.
Financial Disincentives	• Locally adjusted fee schedules for clinical research tasks, to compensate practitioners; • Private payer support, modeled on Medicare program, to provide "coverage with evidence development" (CED) for novel treatments; and • Funding support for clinical trials by employers concerned about health care–related costs.

SOURCE: This table is based on comments made by individuals participating in workshop discussions and the presentation of the Discussion Paper: Eisenberg et al, 2012. *Developing a Clinical Trials Infrastructure*. Discussion Paper, Institute of Medicine. (See Appendix G.)

6

Suggesting an Agenda for Transforming Elements of the Clinical Trials Enterprise

A wrap-up session concluded the workshop and included interpretive summary reports by the chairs of each of the four previous sessions, a panel discussion in which panelists considered elements of an agenda for a transformed CTE, and an open discussion among panelists and audience participants oriented around key questions identified by the workshop planning committee. CTE transformation could substantially benefit several types of stakeholders, for whom such transformation is a shared responsibility:

- patients and families;
- health professionals, including community practitioners;
- hospitals and integrated health delivery systems;
- public and private payers;
- pharmaceutical and medical device manufacturers; and
- the community of investigators, funding organizations, and regulatory agencies engaged in, supporting, or evaluating clinical research.

The chairs of the workshop sessions delivered summaries of their respective discussions. The summaries and workshop discussions generated several key themes on the need for, and possible avenues for transforming, the CTE. Box 6-1 displays these themes. The information in Box 6-1 provides an integrated summary of their remarks and discussions during the panel and should not be construed as reflecting consensus or

BOX 6-1
Key Themes of Clinical Trials Enterprise Transformation
Suggested at the Workshop

This box provides an integrated summary of presentations by Alastair Wood, Professor of Medicine and Pharmacology, Weill Cornell Medical College, and Symphony Capital LLC; Sherine Gabriel, William J. and Charles H. Mayo Professor of Medicine and Epidemiology, Mayo Medical School; Arthur Rubenstein, Professor of Medicine, Division of Endocrinology, Raymond and Ruth Perelman School of Medicine, University of Pennsylvania; and Clyde Yancy, Chief of Cardiology, Northwestern University Feinberg School of Medicine, and Associate Director, Bluhm Cardiovascular Institute, Northwestern Memorial Hospital. These speakers were asked to summarize and discuss key themes arising from their respective sessions of the workshop.

Convergence of Clinical Research and Clinical Practice
* Incorporate clinical research and clinical trials into continuous quality improvement activities of the health care system. Most clinical decisions apparently are not yet based on scientific evidence; broad engagement of, and partnership with, community health care providers and patients could provide excellent opportunities to generate valid, reliable, and relevant evidence and incorporate it into medical practice.
* Focus clinical trials on answering important health questions likely to draw greater interest and support from patients, the public, practitioners, and payers.
* Design less bureaucratic platforms for studies, using EHRs maintained in routine care and novel ways of randomizing patients. Different treatments and populations will give rise to the need for different approaches.
* Expand research networks and collaborate with professional societies in order to centralize processes and induce more physicians to participate in research. Strive to reduce the large footprint on clinical practice that research imposes; research will become part of routine practice only if it is not overly cumbersome.

Workforce and Career Development
* Ensure that those who develop clinical trials examine trial proposals from the perspective of a scientist, as well as from the patient perspective in order to understand what an appropriate and meaningful clinical trial would look like for patients and society.
* Greater diversity in the research workforce would help respond to changing U.S. demographics.
* Secondary education may be an effective venue for educating the public about scientific evidence and beginning to attract young people to careers in science.
* More attention to research in medical schools could improve practitioners' attitudes toward research and attract young physicians to research careers. Innovations in education and training to prepare researchers to collaborate with clinicians could lead to better trials.
* Build education programs—prelicensure, graduate, and lifelong learning—on needs assessments that take into account knowledge gaps, research methodology, interpretation of results, implementation of findings, design thinking, team leadership skills, and business skills.
* Place a higher value on clinical trials research in tenure decisions could enhance CTE career ladders.

Public Engagement and Partnership
- Recognize patients as partners in transforming clinical trials. Consider virtual clinical trial models that use mobile and web-based technologies to conduct clinical trials so that participation in a clinical trial is not dictated by geographic proximity to a trial site.
- Engage the public in order to obtain sufficient and sustained support of the CTE, through both participation in trials and general recognition of the value of clinical research.
- The public and policy makers often do not see how research leads to better outcomes and savings. Creating national awareness of the linkages between clinical research, medical breakthroughs, and ultimately improvements in patient care will require effective communication strategies developed in partnership with the clinical research community and the public.
- Consider implementation of a default consent or "opt-out" process for participation in some types of clinical research. Default consent would create a legal presumption that the patient agrees to allow use of his or her deidentified record for research purposes.
- Undertake communication efforts to the public by the research community to pave the way for direct-to-patient research and the use of social media to recruit individuals into community-based models of research, perhaps eventually supplanting the traditional academic model of Phase III clinical trials.
- Involve patients, the public, practitioners, and payers (including, for example, pharmacy benefit managers) more heavily in conversations about CTE transformation. A new lexicon may be needed to facilitate communication between researchers and the public.

Regulatory Environment
- Improve understanding and communication between government regulators and research organizations.
- Ease the regulatory environment when appropriate, in order to reduce the duration and cost of trials and make them more feasible, especially in domestic settings.
- Update the Common Rule to facilitate fit-for-purpose, patient-friendly repositories of patient data and randomized research projects, especially involving biomarkers and the development of personalized medicine.

Cultural and Financial Incentives
- Undertake the "creative destruction" of old clinical trial business models in favor of newer business models that complement advances in technology.
- Encourage academic health and science centers and research organizations to move beyond provincial systems in favor of greater efficiency for the CTE (e.g., legacy systems, such as site-specific IRBs in favor of using a centralized IRB model).
- Create template contracts to streamline collaborations and subcontracts.
- Consider the role of CMS in CTE transformation. Should tasks associated with bridging the divide between clinical research and clinical practice become a component of Accountable Care Organizations (ACOs)? Should new incentives be created to spur the sustained and collaborative participation of ACOs in research?
- Correct disincentives for research, by using more coverage under evidence development (by private payers as well as Medicare) and reimbursing the routine care costs of research participants.

endorsement by the workshop participants, the planning committee, the Forum, or the National Academies.

Several participants expressed the view that, to spur transformation by 2020, it would be advantageous to move from discussion to action quickly. Patience is needed, however, as each major step along the way is likely to be measured in terms of years. Clyde Yancy, Northwestern University, noted a few issues raised during the discussion on the clinical trials infrastructure:

- Who pays, and how much? The ideas suggested at the workshop will generate substantial costs.
- How can poorly designed trials be avoided?
- Which regulatory objectives should be relaxed in order to reduce the regulatory burden on clinical research?
- Who is liable for adverse events in globalized research?
- Who owns aggregated patient care data, and what rights or privileges does ownership entail?

REFLECTING ON POTENTIAL PATHS FORWARD

It is a huge opportunity to . . . harness a new level of interest in a lot of organizations that would have never thought collectively about participating in research.
—*Douglas Cropper, Genesis Health Systems*

Perspectives on developing an agenda for CTE transformation were offered by Douglas Cropper, President and CEO, Genesis Health Systems; Lynn Etheredge, Independent Consultant on health care and social policy issues, and Head, Rapid Learning Project, The George Washington University; Ronald Krall, Associate Fellow, University of Pennsylvania Center for Bioethics; James Doroshow, Director, Division of Cancer Treatment and Diagnosis, National Cancer Institute (NCI), NIH; and Jean Rouleau, Scientific Director, Institute of Circulatory and Respiratory Health, Canadian Institutes of Health and Research.

A Health Delivery Systems Perspective[1]

Collaboration across community-based systems of care could substantially enhance the CTE infrastructure. Although such collaboration would represent something of a departure from existing practice, because

---

[1] This section is based on the presentation by Douglas Cropper, President and CEO, Genesis Health Systems. Genesis is a six-hospital system in the Quad Cities area of Iowa and Illinois.

the health care system is currently undergoing a great deal of change, many current practices are able to be reconsidered. Much of the change is caused by new incentives. Payers are starting to gear payment levels to value rather than volume and are prodding providers to assume risk for the health of the populations they serve. These payment changes make use of best practices that undergird the provision of adequately reimbursed care.

Other actions by payers also could facilitate further development of a learning health system. Just as federal "meaningful use" incentives are driving health systems nationwide to adopt EHRs more rapidly, so could Medicare be used to create incentives for providers to use EHRs for research (not just to make care more efficient and easily monitored) and to help determine ways to connect data repositories.

CEOs of health systems have been a largely untapped resource in promoting clinical research. Box 6-2 suggests ways health system leadership can serve transformation of the CTE. Engaging this group of leaders can be accomplished by appealing to their business and clinical interests.

BOX 6-2[a]
CEOs of Integrated Health Systems
Could Promote Clinical Research

Health system CEOs could play a crucial role in transformation of the CTE. This role might include

- acting assertively to embed research in the mission and culture of the health system, creating opportunities for the pursuit of scientific evidence within clinical care in order to improve quality, and moving their organizations in the direction of becoming learning health systems (as discussed in Chapter 2);
- promoting clinician training in research (as discussed in Chapter 3);
- facilitating research projects, partly by creating incentives for clinicians to engage in research (as discussed in Chapter 4) and by providing seed grants for health professionals to pursue their research interests; and
- joining research collaboratives or networks on behalf of their organizations (as discussed in Chapter 5).

---

[a] This box is based on the presentation by Douglas Cropper, President and CEO, Genesis Health Systems.

A Health Sciences Policy Perspective[2]

A high-performance clinical research system would produce and disseminate research results on a timely basis. Such a system would encompass more than clinical trials, which—although growing in importance and perhaps volume—will occupy only a portion of the clinical research universe. Box 6-3 lists some of the changes that could take place as the new high-performance clinical research system emerges. Today's data-poor environment would yield to one that is rich with data about virtually all patients and all health conditions, collected through repositories, registries, and networks. The availability of these data would enable a continuous cycle of quality improvement. Participation would be a matter of course, instead of a matter of exception, and clinicians, too, would routinely engage in research. Data silos would disappear. The change could be global in scope.

As part of this change, the CTE would begin to look like other twenty-first century areas of science, such as physics, where there is a European Organization for Nuclear Research, or CERN, which is now leading the search for the Standard Model Higgs boson (CERN, 2011; Vastag and Achenbach, 2011). This means the CTE would rely more on observational studies and predictive models and less on experiments that compare limited, or even ineffective, uses of specific molecules. Such experimentation, after all, is more suited to a slow learning system than a rapid one.

Although public and private payers are attempting to promote the use of research results and scientific evidence in clinical practice, today's clinical effectiveness evidence base is too small, according to Etheredge. Large payers—Medicare especially—have the capacity to collect data on very large populations and use the data to steer clinical practice in more effective directions. To this end, Medicare has established the Partnership for Patients (a public–private venture to prevent unnecessary complications of care, such as hospital-acquired infections), with an eye toward creating more demand by patients and providers for better evidence. This represents a strategy shift from "push" to "pull" in promoting change.

To generate and use data on a far larger scale, and consistently, will require a new technology learning system, in which payers support a research plan for each clinical issue that arises, such as how and when to use a new drug or device. It also will require a new payment system, which bases reimbursement on adherence to evidence-based guidelines that result from research. Then, payers will be able to pay for care that has been shown to be safe and effective. Providers would compete on the basis of quality, determined through proven measures.

---

[2] This subsection is based on a presentation by Lynn Etheredge, Independent Consultant on health care and social policy issues, and Head, Rapid Learning Project, The George Washington University.

BOX 6-3[a]
Aspects of a High-Performance Clinical Research System

A clinical research system that generates, disseminates, and supports the use of scientific findings on a timely basis could have several distinguishing features or characteristics:

- Outcomes data would exist on the great bulk of patients and health conditions and would be shared through data repositories, registries, and networks.
- These data would drive continuous quality improvement for health care providers generally.
- People and health professionals would routinely engage in the research process.
- The transformed clinical research system would even collect data from other countries and could inform health care globally.
- The clinical research system would be more predictive and observational and less experimentally based. In this respect it would move closer to other fields of science.
- Public and private payers, especially Medicare, would use their patient care databases to construct useful evidence about the effectiveness of treatments and other health care interventions.
- A new technology system would link a specific research plan to the rise of each new health care product and modality, to ensure the development of timely findings to inform how and when the product or modality will be used.
- A new payment system would reward quality, based on adherence to evidence-based care. Providers would compete on quality.

---

[a] This box is based on the presentation by Lynn Etheredge, Independent Consultant on health care and social policy issues, and Head, Rapid Learning Project, The George Washington University.

A Research Organization Perspective[3]

The capacity of the CTE, in terms of time, money, and patient participation, is inadequate to efficiently conduct the number of trials that are currently initiated. By one analysis using ClinicalTrials.gov data, clinical trials today call for the enrollment of 1 in every 200 Americans as study participants (IOM, 2010a). In addition, it has been suggested many of the trials being conducted today are of low quality or provide a questionable contribution to advancing knowledge of medicine or health care. A number of workshop participants indicated an interest in systematically

---

[3] This section is based on the presentation by Ronald Krall, Associate Fellow, University of Pennsylvania Center for Bioethics.

studying the quality of clinical trials submitted to the ClinicalTrials.gov registry to validate or refute the impression of generally low quality clinical trials.

Given the concerns with the capacity and quality of the CTE, the question was posed: Should the nation's research portfolio be managed, or should it continue to evolve naturally? A managed approach would help ensure that clinical research, a scarce resource, is used efficiently, with the highest priority being assigned to the most important clinical questions. Under a managed approach, central managers or key decision makers could help ensure that trials meet high scientific standards, if this central authority had authority to deny funding for proposed studies of inferior quality. Management also could help ensure that research results are used systematically to improve care. How would management occur? Box 6-4 displays some alternative ways in which decisions in managing the CTE could be made.

An NIH Perspective[4]

Involving a full range of stakeholders—patient advocacy organizations, participants in trials, professional associations, regulatory agencies, and others—in strategic decision making, while time-consuming, is valuable and appropriate. Box 6-5 contains reflections offered by Doroshow on the need for NIH to relate effectively to patient advocates.

In pursuing change, NIH has achieved some key small successes, and small successes can create momentum for a deeper transformation. The NIH successes have included some achievements by the NCI, which, taken together, have had the effect of reorganizing the NCI clinical trial system.[5] These achievements include

- reducing the length of time for initiating clinical trials;
- centralizing IRB review;
- streamlining the process for gaining access to INDs and obtaining investigational device exemptions;

---

[4] This section is based on the presentation by James Doroshow, Director, Division of Cancer Treatment and Diagnosis, NCI, NIH.

[5] Also of note is NCI's Provocative Questions initiative, which provides an opportunity for investigators to propose intriguing questions in cancer research that need attention but would usually find it difficult to get. The initiative has drawn participation from investigators from a wide range of scientific disciplines and career stages to develop well-conceived, yet provocative, scientific questions in cancer research. NCI has set aside $15 million from the 2012 budget to support new grants for the best ideas to answer the provocative questions that have been developed (Varmus and Harlow, 2012). For more information visit http://provocativequestions.nci.nih.gov/ (accessed March 28, 2012).

BOX 6-4[a]
Possible Ways to Manage the
Research Portfolio in the United States

- By a *formally convened panel of stakeholders* that applies explicit standards, based on a utilitarian criterion of the greatest benefit to the greatest number of people and (to a lesser extent) a cost criterion of the greatest potential savings;
- Through a *market model*, as health plans, IHSs, or people themselves decide which studies to participate in, and only studies drawing enough support are conducted; or
- In "*shining the light*" on individual decisions, by using social media to let people vote their preferences among possible studies.

These approaches are not mutually exclusive and could be combined as appropriate. For example, a narrow set of research questions of great importance to population health could be determined by an expert committee, a market approach could be applied to remaining research questions, and a "shine the light" approach could overlay the entire research portfolio.

---

[a] This box is based on the presentation by Ronald Krall, Associate Fellow, University of Pennsylvania Center for Bioethics.

BOX 6-5[a]
One NIH Official's Reflections on
Collaborating with Patient Advocates

I have learned a great deal about advocacy and the role of advocates. And while it sometimes can be difficult to satisfy the needs of all of the advocates across all of the disease entities that are represented in the diseases that the NCI provides support for its clinical trials, it has really been remarkably important. Because advocates represent patients, and patients are not satisfied with the status quo. And they really have pushed, and they have pushed very hard, for us to do things differently, to do things more effectively, to do things much, much faster. And [they] have not allowed us to settle in.

---

[a] This quote is from James Doroshow, Director, Division of Cancer Treatment and Diagnosis, NCI, NIH.

- decentralizing the process for prioritizing research areas;
- implementing a new trials data management system, with specifications designed primarily by investigators;
- certifying imaging sites and radiation therapy programs for quality control, so that results of studies conducted at different sites can be reliably compared;
- enhancing core clinical laboratories, so that laboratory tests in different trials will have the same platforms;
- creating the NCI Clinical Investigator Team Leadership Award, to promote genomic research by providing small grants to younger researchers; and
- reforming the NCI network, to support an increased level of grant support.

An International Perspective[6]

Canada, like the United States, faces the twin problems of developing a scientific evidence base for clinical care and constraining health care costs. Health expenditures account for 11 percent of Canada's gross domestic product (compared with 18 percent in the United States) and the rate of increase in expenditures is considered unsustainable. In response, the Canadian Institutes of Health and Research has spearheaded an effort to promote the development, translation, and use of "patient-oriented research." Box 6-6 shows components of the strategy underlying this effort. Key features of the strategy include citizen engagement and partnerships with stakeholders (such as academic institutions and life science industries), comprehensiveness in addressing all types of obstacles to clinical research (such as biostatistics and infrastructure), and a focus on improving quality and containing costs.

A national task force might be an effective vehicle for creating the organizational underpinning of CTE transformation in the United States, suggested Rouleau. Other suggestions included streamlining regulations, involving young scientists and clinicians in designing education and training initiatives, helping academic health and science centers develop research networks, integrating research data and EHRs through a new business model, promoting adaptive research designs such as cluster trials, sponsoring "research on research," and participating in international collaborations.

---

[6] This section is based on the presentation by Jean Rouleau, Scientific Director, Institute of Circulatory and Respiratory Health, Canadian Institutes of Health and Research.

BOX 6-6^a
Components of the Canadian Strategy for
Patient-Oriented Research

- *Improve the research environment and infrastructure,* through research networks, beginning with primary care and mental health, and through provincially based support units on data management, project management, and other aspects of studies.
- *Set up mechanisms to better train and mentor health professionals and non-clinicians in health research,* through career paths established by partnerships with organizations that fund relevant education and training programs.
- *Strengthen organizational, regulatory, and financial support for multisite studies,* through provincial ethics review panels, a national template for contracts, national cost and operations standards, a simplified procedure for reporting adverse events, common databases, and common EHRs.
- *Support best practices in health care,* through knowledge transfer to patients.

---

[a] This box is based on the presentation by Jean Rouleau, Scientific Director, Institute of Circulatory and Respiratory Health, Canadian Institutes of Health and Research.

BUILDING A FRAMEWORK AND SUGGESTING AN AGENDA

We need to pay for things that are safe and effective. We need to
stop paying for things that are not safe and effective.
—Lynn Etheredge, The George Washington University

The workshop's concluding discussion was oriented around six questions presented to workshop participants:

1. *Long-term goals:* What are the long-term strategic goals that we need to identify and meet?
2. *Priorities:* What are the top three priorities for reform, based on their urgency, scope, and/or importance to the transformation effort?
3. *Short-term goals:* What are the top three to five opportunities that represent "low-hanging fruit" or are realistic short-term goals for improving the productivity and effectiveness of our CTE?
4. *Workforce:* What are key opportunities and strategies for developing and leveraging a workforce to support the CTE?
5. *Infrastructure:* How can disease and patient advocacy networks, voluntary health associations, and other nongovernmental and

nonprofit organizations contribute to or coordinate efforts to build an infrastructure for clinical trials?

6. *Stakeholder engagement:* How do we build an agenda through the following stakeholder groups: (a) health care delivery systems; (b) the pharmaceutical and biotech industries; (c) payers; (d) disease and patient advocacy networks, voluntary health associations, and other nongovernmental and nonprofit organizations; (e) the education and training enterprise, including academic health and science centers; and (f) regulators and federal agencies that fund or support research?

Workshop chair Jeffrey Drazen, *New England Journal of Medicine*, led the discussion.

The next subsection summarizes individual participants' suggestions responding to questions 1-4. The subsection after that summarizes individual participants' suggestions responding to questions 5 and 6. It should not be construed as reflecting consensus or endorsement by the workshop participants, the planning committee, the Forum, or the National Academies.

Building an Agenda, Establishing a Framework

What are the long-term strategic goals that we need to identify and meet?

Among possible long-term goals mentioned by individual participants were

- *moving research "into the community"* by enlisting greater participation by community practitioners, partly through leverage exerted by leaders of IHSs. Together with making research "business-critical" or "mission-critical"—making research an essential component of the work of IHSs and other large providers of care—a community focus could greatly help align the CTE and the health system;
- *greater regulatory harmonization and simplification,* especially with regard to IRBs; and
- *routinely enrolling people newly diagnosed with key chronic diseases, such as diabetes, into clinical trials.* The clinician plays a pivotal role in recruitment at the point of care and can partner with the patient to determine if participation in a clinical trial is in her or his best interest.

Moving the CTE "into the community" and routinely enrolling newly diagnosed people into trials could improve the utility of research, increase

---

BOX 6-7[a]
Public Engagement in Clinical Trials

Public engagement in clinical trials may include obtaining more public input into decisions about which topics to study and about the actual designs of studies, including clinical end points (that is, the measurable outcome that denotes a successful treatment). This could happen through several means, including a type of online voting or discussion, structured involvement by patient-oriented advocacy groups, and training of community health leaders.

Public engagement also could be linked to formal public education. Patients and citizens may be most likely to engage in trials if they become aware that a great deal of new research is needed to ensure that people receive care that will help them. And, public education could have the best chance of creating an impact if it is undertaken through a formal strategy, rather than by relying on the news media and social media.

---

[a]This box is based on remarks by John Gallin, Director, NIH Clinical Center; Janet Tobias, CEO, Ikana Health; Annetine Gelijns, Co-Chair, Department of Health Evidence and Policy, Mount Sinai School of Medicine; and Heather Snyder, Senior Associate Director for Scientific Grants, Alzheimer's Association International Research Grant Program, and workshop discussions.

---

participation rates, and enhance public support for clinical research in general.[7] Box 6-7 describes some possible features of such public engagement. The specific suggestion of allowing the public to "vote with their feet" to choose which areas to study (see the description of the market model in Box 6-3) received support from some workshop participants as a way to root the research enterprise in communities, but it also was criticized as unrealistic, partly because most patients typically are not educated to evaluate trial designs and methods.

What are the top three priorities for reform, based on their urgency, scope, and/or importance to the transformation effort?

In pursuit of these goals, possible priorities mentioned by individual participants were

---

[7] The NIH launched a new website, "NIH Clinical Research Trials and You," with user-friendly information on what clinical trials are, why they matter, and how an individual can get involved (http://www.nih.gov/health/clinicaltrials/index.htm [accessed March 28, 2012]). The website also includes resources for health care providers, drawn from successful approaches used in pediatric oncology, to help them discuss with patients the possibility of enrolling in a clinical trial.

- education of patients, health professionals (including the use of continuing education), and payers;
- incentives for research, perhaps informed by research into how other industries have developed thriving and sustainable systems of research and development; and
- adoption of the proposed revisions to the Common Rule.[8]

Education could include educating practitioners about clinical research and defining the attributes of a good, or at least internally valid, study. But education alone is not likely to suffice in bringing about reform. A theme mentioned several times during the workshop is that transformation of the CTE requires a shifting of the incentives that payers impose on providers of care—namely, a shift away from procedures and volume and toward value, population health, and quality of care, as determined through scientific evidence.

What are the top three to five opportunities that represent "low-hanging fruit" or are realistic short-term goals for improving the productivity and effectiveness of our CTE?

Realistic short-term goals for CTE improvement identified by individual participants include

- making the health IT systems of most providers of care interoperable;
- simplifying the IRB process, through ways suggested in Box 6-8;
- exempting low-risk research (e.g., quality improvement initiatives, research conducted by surveys) from the traditional regulatory and administrative burdens on research, such as the IRB process;
- HHS development of "work plans" on specific research questions, with time-limited, open competition for other researchers to develop better, cheaper, or faster ways to answer the same question;
- standardizing the clinical trials nomenclature (harmonization of the concepts that are universal across clinical trials but have different names currently in use);
- improvements in the ClinicalTrials.gov process, such as entering of more and better data by trial registrants[9] or making website contents subject to editing or oversight;

---

[8] See Chapter 5, footnote 4, and surrounding text.

[9] Timely reporting of trial results on ClinicalTrials.gov has been found inadequate by one study. According to a study of 40,000 trials registered on the site between 1999 and 2010, only 12 percent reported results within the required 1 year of completion of the trial. Late reporting, say the study authors, "is troublesome and may affect the overall usefulness of the registry in expanding clinical knowledge in a timely manner." The study further found

---

BOX 6-8
Individual Workshop Participants' Suggestions for
Simplifying the IRB Process

- Centralizing IRB functions within IHSs and other large research organizations, perhaps by creating "super IRBs";
- Avoiding overly long informed consent forms that discourage would-be participants;
- Improving consistency in how different IRBs interpret the standard questions in the basic IRB application form; and
- Reducing regulatory requirements for non-research-related uses of data, such as quality improvement or reporting of medical errors.

- engaging more health care system CEOs in clinical research, perhaps incorporating "clinical research" within the framework of "quality improvement" or "best practices" in order to demystify it; and
- creating a national, publicly accessible roster of clinical researchers (similar to what has been done at NCI recently).

These achievements were seen as "small wins" that could create momentum for change.

What are key opportunities and strategies for developing and leveraging a workforce to support the CTE?

According to several workshop participants, a key workforce-related strategy is the creation and maintenance of vibrant and continually energized research networks. These networks could be organized around specific diseases, other discrete health issues, or alliances of IHSs. Networks could provide ongoing credentialing or engagement of researchers, so that a new team—sometimes with less-skilled members—does not have to be recruited, trained, and approved for each new study.

---

that the number of registered trials declined steadily after 2008 and, by January 2010, had fallen to the same level in place before the federal mandate to register all clinical trials took effect. Yet, no penalties for noncompliance with the mandate were issued as of February 2010 (Law et al., 2011). (The mandate was part of the 2007 FDA Amendments Act and applies to all Phase II and higher trials conducted in the United States or as part of the FDA's IND application process.)

Building an Agenda, by Stakeholder

How can disease and patient advocacy networks, voluntary health associations, and other nongovernmental and nonprofit organizations contribute to or coordinate efforts to build an infrastructure for clinical trials?

Ways to enhance the roles of advocacy groups, in the views of various individual participants, include

- expanding public education about clinical research, so patients and families are better prepared to support research efforts;
- promoting the Health Research Alliance, a consortium of organizations supporting clinical research, as a site for "one-stop shopping" for research organizations seeking to collaborate with voluntary and advocacy associations; and
- encouraging groups representing patients and families to use the CF community, the multiple myeloma community, and people with HIV/AIDS as some of the models for promoting a vigorous research agenda and obtaining a high level of participation in trials.

Advocacy groups, an individual participant noted, are moving toward direct sponsorship of studies, forsaking their previous "hands-off" approach to research. Advocates tend to be supportive of the role of pharmaceutical, biotech, and medical device research and manufacturing firms, while occasionally criticizing academic health and science centers, private third-party payers, and authors of regulations, and so the latter entities could benefit from working to improve these relationships.

How do we build an agenda through the following stakeholder groups: (a) health care delivery systems; (b) the pharmaceutical and biotech industries; (c) payers; (d) disease and patient advocacy networks, voluntary health associations, and other nongovernmental and nonprofit organizations; (e) the education and training enterprise, including academic health and science centers; and (f) regulators and federal agencies that fund or support research?

Table 6-1 lists ideas presented by the panelists and workshop participants. Statements, recommendations, and opinions expressed are those of individual presenters and participants and are not necessarily endorsed or verified by the Forum or the National Academies, and they should not be construed as reflecting any group consensus.

TABLE 6-1 Illustrative Strategies for Action by Stakeholder Groups Suggested by Individual Workshop Participants

Stakeholder Group	Possible Strategies to Advance CTE Transformation Suggested by Individual Workshop Participants
Health care delivery systems	• Build research into quality improvement programs and strive for cultural change as a business opportunity; • Enlist CEOs to lead local public education efforts; • Develop research business plans, and adapt to a new business model; and • Use EHRs for research.
Pharmaceutical and biotech firms	• Reduce outsourcing of studies (to ensure their applicability to the U.S. population); • Create a standing research capacity with an IHS partner as a demonstration project; and • Use new research approaches, e.g., cluster randomization, pragmatic trials, adaptive designs, and virtual trials.
Public and private third-party payers	• Implementation by CMS of research conclusions, especially in coverage with evidence development (CED); • Cover study participants' medical costs and community practitioners' research work; • Use more value-based insurance design, incorporating scientific evidence; and • Increase involvement in research, such as by suggesting studies.
Advocacy networks and voluntary associations	• Advance public education of clinical research to engage the public as part of the CTE workforce; • Develop new and stronger consortia and research alliances; and • Increase involvement in research, such as by contributing to study designs.
Academic health and science centers and educators	• Match new graduate researchers with projects that will generate results, and assign them to mentors; • Foster research as part of health professions curricula; • Build five-tier system of workforce development (public, community practitioners, implementers, investigators, methodologists), with demographic diversity; • Promote elementary and secondary school education on research; • Include research questions on professional licensing and board exams; and • Use online training for research project staff.

continued

TABLE 6-1 Continued

Stakeholder Group	Possible Strategies to Advance CTE Transformation Suggested by Individual Workshop Participants
Regulators and federal agencies that support research	• Enhance collaboration in developing the learning health system among NIH, FDA, and other HHS components, with overarching attention by the HHS Secretary to clinical research; • Make large databases accessible to researchers, with registries online; • Place the organization of CER efforts under the purview of the HHS Secretary; • Develop more public–private research partnerships; and • Relax principal investigator requirement, harmonize regulations, show greater flexibility, and promulgate regulatory "safe harbors."

Illustrative actions that could be taken by all stakeholder groups include the following suggestions made during the course of the workshop:

- strengthening the "four labs" of innovation, traditional, health care delivery, and community engagement;
- agreeing on national leadership of the CTE;
- establishing a national research agenda, to be reviewed and modified every several years;
- creating a central data repository, to merge treatment results from all providers;
- merging research organizations' information systems on compliance and preparing standard contracts, to reduce study costs; and
- creating a standard international nomenclature, to make study results from different countries compatible.

Moving, within one decade, from relatively few decisions being evidence-based to nearly all decisions being evidence-based—and being entered into a researchable database—will require traversing a great distance. Individual workshop participants variously mentioned at least five discrete steps that could be applied to each medical treatment or intervention: (1) Results of previous experience with the treatment or intervention could be obtained (through clinical trials or observational data) for sufficient numbers of patients in order to permit valid statistical analyses of the treatment's efficacy or effectiveness; (2) demographic, disease, and biologic factors affecting the success of the treatment could be identified; (3) a protocol could be developed for applying these research results to the care of individual patients; (4) the bulk of clinicians could use the protocol when appropriate; and (5) patients and families would understand the advantages of evidence-based care, participate in the studies necessary for medical advances, and join with clinicians in demanding clinical care that is based on medical evidence. The foundation of all these steps is the CTE.

References

Adams, C. P., and V. V. Brantner. 2006. Estimating the cost of new drug development: Is it really $802 million? *Health Affairs* 25(2):420-428. http://content.healthaffairs.org/content/25/2/420.full.html (accessed January 31, 2012).

AHRQ (Agency for Healthcare Research and Quality). 2011. *AHRQ at a glance.* http://www.ahrq.gov/about/ataglance.htm (accessed November 11, 2011).

Bonham, A. C., R. M. Califf, E. K. Gallin, and M. S. Lauer. 2012. *Developing a robust clinical trials workforce.* Discussion Paper, Institute of Medicine, Washington, DC.

Califf, R. M., G. L. Filerman, R. K. Murray, and M. Rosenblatt. 2012. *The clinical trials enterprise in the United States: A call for disruptive innovation.* Discussion Paper, Institute of Medicine, Washington, DC.

CenterWatch. 2011. *Proposed Common Rule updates focus on consent, definitions, streamlined IRB review, data protection.* October 31. http://centerwatch.com/news-online/article/2443/proposed-common-rule-updates-focus-on-consent-definitions-streamlined-irb-review-data-protection (accessed January 11, 2012).

CERN (European Organization for Nuclear Research). 2011. *ATLAS and CMS experiments present Higgs search status.* http://public.web.cern.ch/public/ (accessed December 18, 2011).

DeVol, R. C., A. Bedroussian, and B. Yeo. 2011. *The global biomedical industry: Preserving U.S. leadership.* http://www.milkeninstitute.org/pdf/CASMIFullReport.pdf (accessed February 9, 2012).

Deyell, M.W., C. E. Buller, L. H. Miller, T. Y. Wang, D. Dai, G. A. Lamas, V. S. Srinivas, and J. S. Hochman. 2011. Impact of National Clinical Guideline recommendations for revascularization of persistently occluded infarct-related arteries on clinical practice in the United States. *Archives of Internal Medicine* 171(18):1636-1643.

Dzau, V. J., D. C. Ackerly, P. Sutton-Wallace, M. H. Merson, R. S. Williams, K. R. Krishnan, R. C. Taber, and R. M. Califf. 2010. The role of academic health science systems in the transformation of medicine. *Lancet* 375:949-953.

Eisenberg, P., P. Kaufmann, E. V. Sigal, and J. Woodcock. 2012. *Developing a clinical trials infrastructure.* Discussion Paper, Institute of Medicine, Washington, DC.

Executive Office of the President, President's Council of Advisors on Science and Technology. 2010. *Realizing the full potential of health information technology to improve healthcare for Americans: The path forward.* Report to the President. Washington, DC: The White House. http://www.whitehouse.gov/sites/default/files/microsites/ostp/pcast-health-it-report. pdf (accessed November 10, 2011).

FDA (Food and Drug Administration). 2010. *Advancing regulatory science for public health.* http://www.fda.gov/ScienceResearch/SpecialTopics/RegulatoryScience/ucm228131. htm (accessed January 23, 2012).

Gallin, J. I. 2011. *Sustaining institutional support and patient engagement in clinical trials: Models and messages from the NIH Clinical Center.* Speaker presentation at the IOM Workshop on Envisioning a Transformed Clinical Trials Enterprise in the United States: Establishing an Agenda for 2020, November 7, Washington, DC.

HHS (Department of Health and Human Services). 2011. *Advanced Notice of Proposed Rulemaking: Human subjects protections update.* http://www.hhs.gov/ohrp/humansubjects/ index.html (accessed December 12, 2011).

Hochman, J. S., G. A. Lamas, C. E. Buller, H. Dzavik, H. R. Reynolds, S. J. Abramsky, S. Forman, W. Ruzyllo, A. P. Maggioni, H. White, Z. Sadowski, A. C. Carvalho, J. M. Rankin, J. P. Renkin, P. G. Steg, A. M. Mascette, G. Sopko, M. E. Pfisterer, J. Leor, V. Fridrich, D. B. Mark, and G. L. Knatterud. 2006. Coronary intervention for persistent occlusion after myocardial infarction. *New England Journal of Medicine* 355(23):2395-2407.

i2b2. 2011. *Informatics for integrating biology and the bedside.* https://www.i2b2.org/ (accessed December 2, 2011).

IOM (Institute of Medicine). 2001. *Crossing the quality chasm: A new health system for the 21st century.* Washington, DC: National Academy Press.

IOM. 2004. *Health literacy: A prescription to end confusion.* Washington, DC: The National Academies Press.

IOM. 2007. *The learning healthcare system. Workshop summary.* Washington, DC: The National Academies Press.

IOM. 2009. *Initial national priorities for comparative effectiveness research.* Washington, DC: The National Academies Press.

IOM. 2010a. *Transforming clinical research in the United States: Challenges and opportunities. Workshop summary.* Washington, DC: The National Academies Press.

IOM. 2010b. *The healthcare imperative: Lowering costs and improving outcomes. Workshop summary.* Washington, DC: The National Academies Press.

IOM. 2011a. *Engineering a learning healthcare system: A look at the future. Workshop summary.* Washington, DC: The National Academies Press.

IOM. 2011b. *Learning what works: Infrastructure required for comparative effectiveness research. Workshop summary.* Washington, DC: The National Academies Press.

IOM. 2011c. *Innovations in health literacy research. Workshop summary.* Washington, DC: The National Academies Press.

IOM. 2012a. *Public engagement and clinical trials: New models and disruptive technologies. Workshop summary.* Washington, DC: The National Academies Press.

IOM. 2012b. *Strengthening a workforce for innovative regulatory science in therapeutics development. Workshop summary.* Washington, DC: The National Academies Press.

Jolly, M. K. 2011. *PACeR: The Partnership to Accelerate Clinical electronic Research—improves predictive success.* Speaker presentation at the IOM workshop on Envisioning a Transformed Clinical Trials Enterprise in the United States: Establishing an Agenda for 2020, November 8, 2011, Washington, DC.

Kapowich, J. M. 2010. Oregon's test of value-based insurance design in coverage for state workers. *Health Affairs* 29(11):2028-2032.

Kocher, R., and N. R. Sahni. 2011. Rethinking health care labor. *New England Journal of Medicine* 365(15):1370-1372.

Kolodziej, M. A. 2011. The community oncologist: Part of the solution. *Journal of the National Comprehensive Cancer Network* 9:345-347.

Kost, R. G., L. M. Lee, J. Yessis, B. S. Coller, D. K. Henderson, and The Research Participant Perception Survey Focus Group Subcommittee. 2011. Assessing research participants' perceptions of their clinical research experiences. *Clinical and Translational Science* 4(6):403-413.

Kramer, J. M., and K. A. Schulman. 2011. *Transforming the economics of clinical trials.* Speaker presentation at the Institute of Medicine Workshop on Envisioning a Transformed Clinical Trials Enterprise in the United States: Establishing an Agenda for 2020, November 7-8, Washington, DC.

Kramer, J. M., and K. A. Schulman. 2012. *Transforming the economics of clinical trials.* Discussion Paper, Institute of Medicine, Washington, DC.

Law, M. R., Y. Kawasumi, and S. G. Morgan. 2011. Despite law, fewer than one in eight completed studies of drugs and biologics are reported on time on clinicaltrials.gov. *Health Affairs* 30(12):2338-2345.

Lee, D. H., and O. Vielemeyer. 2011. Analysis of overall level of evidence behind Infectious Disease Society of America practice guidelines. *Annals of Internal Medicine* 171:18-22.

Lilford, R. J., and J. Jackson. 1995. Equipoise and the ethics of randomization. *Journal of the Royal Society of Medicine* 88:552-559.

Mackenzie, I. S., L. Wei, D. Rutherford, E. A. Findlay, W. Saywood, M. K. Campbell, and T. M. MacDonald. 2010. Promoting public awareness of randomised clinical trials using the media: The "Get Randomised" campaign. *Journal of Clinical Pharmacology* 69(2):128-135.

Mansell, P. 2011. Pfizer announces "virtual" clinical trial pilot in U.S. *PharmaTimes*, June 9. http://www.pharmatimes.com/Article/11-06-09/Pfizer_announces_virtual_clinical_trial_pilot_in_US.aspx (accessed December 8, 2011).

National Marfan Foundation. 2011. *Atenolol versus losartan clinical trial.* http://www.marfan.org/marfan/2408/Atenolol-vs.-Losartan-Clinical-Trial (accessed December 5, 2011).

NIH (National Institutes of Health), Division of Program Coordination, Planning and Strategic Initiatives. 2011. *The NIH Common Fund.* http://commonfund.nih.gov/researchteams/index.aspx (accessed November 18, 2011).

NIH, Scientific Management Review Board. 2010. Report on the NIH Clinical Center. http://smrb.od.nih.gov/ (accessed April 10, 2012).

O'Connor, C. M., R. C. Starling, A. F. Hernandez, P. W. Armstrong, K. Dickstein, V. Hasselblad, G. M. Heizer, M. Komajda, B. M. Massie, J. J. V. McMurray, M. S. Nieminen, C. J. Reist, J. L. Rouleau, K. Swedberg, K. F. Adams, S. D. Anker, D. Atar, A. Battler, R. Botero, N. R. Bohidar, J. Butler, N. Clausell, R. Corbalán, M. R. Costanzo, U. Dahlstrom, L. I. Deckelbaum, R. Diaz, M. E. Dunlap, J. A. Ezekowitz, D. Feldman, G. M. Felker, G. C. Fonarow, D. Gennevois, S. S. Gottlieb, J. A. Hill, J. E. Hollander, J. G. Howlett, M. P. Hudson, R. D. Kociol, H. Krum, A. Laucevicius, W. C. Levy, G. F. Méndez, M. Metra, S. Mittal, B.-H. Oh, N. L. Pereira, P. Ponikowski, W. H. W. Tang, S. Tanomsup, J. R. Teerlink, F. Triposkiadis, R. W. Troughton, A. A. Voors, D. J. Whellan, F. Zannad, and R. M. Califf. 2011. Effect of nesiritide in patients with acute decompensated heart failure. *New England Journal of Medicine* 365(1):32-43.

Platt, R., Takvorian S.U., Septimus E., Hickok J., Moody J., Perlin J., Jernigan J. A., Kleinman K., Huang S. S. 2010. Cluster randomized trials in comparative effectiveness research: Randomizing hospitals to test methods for prevention of healthcare-associated infections. *Medical Care* 48(6):S52-S57.

Platt, R., R. M. Carnahan, J. S. Brown, E. Chrischilles, L. H. Curtis, S. Hennessy, J. C. Nelson, J. A. Racoosin, M. Robb, S. Schneeweiss, S. Toh, and M. G. Weiner. 2012. The U.S. Food and Drug Administration's Mini-Sentinel program: Status and direction. *Pharmacoepidemiology and Drug Safety* 21(S1):1-8.

Pollack, A. 2011. FDA approves drug for lupus, an innovation after 50 years. *New York Times*, March 9. http://www.nytimes.com/2011/03/10/health/10drug.html (accessed December 4, 2011).

Ramsey, B. W., J. Davies, N. G. McElvaney, E. Tullis, S. C. Bell, P. Drevinek, M. Griese, E. F. McKone, C. E. Wainwright, M. W. Konstan, R. Moss, F. Ratjen, I. Sermet-Gaudelus, S. M. Rowe, Q. Dong, S. Rodriguez, K. Yen, C. Ordonez, and J. S. Elborn. 2011. A CFTR potentiator in patients with cystic fibrosis and the *G551D* mutation. *New England Journal of Medicine* 365(18):1663-1672.

Research!America. 2007. *Americans expect medical breakthroughs*. http://www.researchamerica.org/uploads/poll.report.2007.transforminghealth.pdf (accessed December 4, 2011).

Rudd, R. E., J. E. Anderson, S. Oppenheimer, and C. Nath. 2007. Health literacy: An update of public health and medical literature. In *Review of Adult Learning and Literacy*, Vol. 7, edited by J. P. Comings, B. Garner, and C. Smith. Mahwah, NJ: Lawrence Erlbaum Associates. Pp. 175-204.

Schaefer, G. O., E. J. Emanuel, and A. Wertheimer. 2009. The obligation to participate in biomedical research. *Journal of the American Medical Association* 302(1):67-72.

Sung, N. S., W. F. Crowley, M. Genel, P. Salber, L. Sandy, L. M. Sherwood, S. B. Johnson, V. Catanese, H. Tilson, K. Getz, E. L. Larson, D. Scheinberg, E. A. Reece, H. Slavkin, A. Dobs, J. Grebb, R. A. Martinez, A. Korn, and D. Rimoin. 2003. Central challenges facing the national clinical research enterprise. *Journal of the American Medical Association* 289(10):1278-1287.

Topol, E.J. 2005. Nesiritide—not verified. *New England Journal of Medicine* 353(2):113-116.

Tricoci, P., J. M. Allen, J. M. Kramer, R. M. Califf, and S. C. Smith, Jr. 2009. Scientific evidence underlying the ACC/AHA clinical practice guidelines. *Journal of the American Medical Association* 301:967-974.

Tufts Center for the Study of Drug Development. 2007. *Impact report: Notable gender and racial disparities exist among clinical investigators*. November/December, 9(6). http://csdd.tufts.edu/files/uploads/08_-_nov._5,_2007_-_principal_investigators.pdf (accessed January 23, 2011).

Varmus, H. and E. Harlow. 2012. Provocative questions in cancer research. *Nature* 481:436-437. http://www.nature.com/nature/journal/v481/n7382/full/481436a.html (accessed January 30, 2012).

Vastag, B., and J. Achenbach. 2011. Scientists close in on linchpin of physics, the "God particle." *Washington Post*, December 12. http://www.washingtonpost.com/national/health-science/scientists-close-in-on-linchpin-of-physics-the-god-particle/2011/12/12/gIQAmk2cqO_story.html (accessed December 18, 2011).

Vincent, G. K., and V. A. Velkoff. 2010. The next four decades: The older population in the United States: 2010 to 2050. *Current Population Reports*. Washington, DC: U.S. Census Bureau.

Wallentin, L., R. C. Becker, A. Budaj, C. P. Cannon, H. Emanuelsson, C. Held, J. Horrow, S. Husted, S. James, H. Katus, K. W. Mahaffey, B. M. Scirica, A. Skene, P. G. Steg, R. F. Storey, and R. A. Harrington. 2009. Ticagrelor versus clopidogrel in patients with acute coronary syndromes. *New England Journal of Medicine* 361(11):1045-1057.

Wood, A. 2011. *Envisioning CTE in the health care system of 2020*. Speaker presentation at the Institute of Medicine Workshop on Envisioning a Transformed Clinical Trials Enterprise in the United States: Establishing an Agenda for 2020, November 7-8, Washington, DC.

Yu, P. 2011. *The learning health system*. Speaker presentation at the IOM workshop on Envisioning a Transformed Clinical Trials Enterprise in the United States: Establishing an Agenda for 2020, November 7, 2011, Washington, DC.

Appendix A

Workshop Agenda

Envisioning a Transformed Clinical Trials Enterprise in the United States: Establishing an Agenda for 2020

November 7-8, 2011

**20 F Street NW Conference Center
20 F Street NW
Washington, DC 20001**

Background:
There is increasing recognition that the clinical trials enterprise in the United States faces substantial challenges impeding the efficient and effective conduct of clinical and translational research needed to support the development of breakthrough medicines. A gap exists between the desired state where medical care in the United States is provided solely based on high-quality evidence and the reality of our limited ability to generate timely and practicable evidence. Eighty-five percent of clinical decisions in the United States are not supported by high-quality evidence. At the same time, U.S. clinical trials that generate medical evidence are becoming increasingly costly while experiencing greater setbacks. In addition, the shifting "footprint" of clinical trials toward sites outside the United States prompts questions about the generalizability and applicability of the results of those clinical trials to the U.S. population and represents a competitive challenge for the United States.

The limited ability of the nation's clinical trials system to support drug development and evaluation exists within a broader context of a need for a "learning health system," where "knowledge generation is so embedded into the core of the practice of medicine that it is a natural outgrowth and product of the health care delivery process and leads to continual improvement in care." An essential component of such a learning health system is a robust and well-working clinical trials enterprise to support drug development; inform quality improvement; and support surveillance, international, and comparative effectiveness research.

The IOM's Forum on Drug Discovery, Development, and Translation has established an initiative to address challenges facing the U.S. clinical trials enterprise and to engage stakeholders in an open discussion of potentially transformative strategies to improve the efficiency and effectiveness of clinical trials.

Workshop Objectives:
- Frame the problem and discuss a vision for a clinical trials enterprise that is efficient and effective and fully integrated into the health delivery system of 2020. Define how the envisioned clinical trials enterprise differs from the current system and suggest approaches to transform our current system into a learning system.
- Consider the following **core themes** in framing an agenda to effect transformation of the U.S. clinical trials enterprise:
  — Providing a vision for a clinical trials enterprise in the health care system of 2020.
  — Developing a robust clinical trials workforce.
  — Aligning cultural and financial incentives.
  — Building an infrastructure to support a transformed clinical trials enterprise.
- Workshop presentations and panel discussions will be supported and supplemented by discussion papers prepared by participants in Forum activities. Each of the four workshop sessions will be prefaced by presentations from discussion paper authors.

NOVEMBER 7, 2011

8:30 a.m.   Breakfast available

9:00 a.m.   Welcome and Introductions

                  JEFFREY DRAZEN, *Workshop Chair*
                  Editor-in-Chief
                  New England Journal of Medicine

SESSION I:
FRAMING THE NEED FOR CHANGE:
ENVISIONING A CLINICAL TRIALS ENTERPRISE
IN THE HEALTH CARE SYSTEM OF 2020

Session Objectives:
- Set a framework within which to establish a vision for 2020 that addresses the reinvention of the clinical trials enterprise around partnership with the institutional health care delivery system of 2020.
- Given the anticipated changes in the structure of the U.S. health care system, consider how an efficient, effective clinical trials enterprise can be integrated into the health care delivery system of 2020.

> ALASTAIR J.J. WOOD, *Session Chair*
> Partner & Managing Director
> Symphony Capital

9:10 a.m.   Presentation of Discussion Paper: *The Clinical Trials Enterprise in the United States: A Call for Disruptive Innovation*

> ROBERT CALIFF
> Director, Duke Translational Medicine Institute
> Professor of Medicine
> Vice Chancellor for Clinical and Translational Research
> Duke University Medical Center

> GARY FILERMAN
> President
> Atlas Health Foundation

> RICHARD MURRAY
> Vice President, Global Center for Scientific Affairs
> Office of the Chief Medical Officer
> Merck & Co., Inc.

10:00 a.m.   **Panel Discussion with Speakers:** *A Framework for the Clinical Trials Enterprise in the Health Care System of 2020*
Objectives:
- Suggest and discuss the key components of a transformed clinical trials enterprise incorporated into the integrated health delivery system of 2020.

- Discuss the research outputs needed from the clinical trials enterprise to drive improved patient care and feed into a learning health system.
- Consider broad transformational changes including the changing shape/structure of the pharmaceutical industry and the increasing globalization in clinical trials and drug development.

  ALASTAIR J.J. WOOD, *Panel Moderator*
  Partner & Managing Director
  Symphony Capital

  NEIL WEISSMAN
  President
  MedStar Health Research Institute

  IHOR RAK
  Vice President, Clinical Neuroscience
  AstraZeneca

10:45 a.m.   BREAK

11:00 a.m.   **Keynote Address:** *The Learning Health System*

  RICHARD PLATT
  Professor, Harvard Medical School
  Co-Chair, Clinical Effectiveness Research Innovation Collaboration
  IOM Roundtable on Value and Science-Driven Health Care

11:30 a.m.   **Discussion with Keynote Speaker, Panelists, and Workshop Participants:**
- How can the national clinical trials enterprise fit into the envisioned learning health system?
- What infrastructure is needed to embed randomized controlled trials in a learning health system?
- What are the key barriers impeding integration of clinical trials into a learning health system (e.g., financial, cultural, regulatory)?
- Where are the opportunities to address these barriers and build the needed infrastructure? What stakeholders/organizations/sectors should take the lead and how can their efforts best be coordinated?

PETER YU, *Moderator*
Oncologist, Palo Alto Medical Foundation
Chair, Electronic Health Record Working Group
American Society of Clinical Oncology

BRYAN LUCE
Senior Vice President, Science Policy
United BioSource Corporation

12:15 p.m.   LUNCH

SESSION II:
DEVELOPING A ROBUST CLINICAL TRIALS WORKFORCE

Session Objectives:
- Define a clinical trials "workforce" and identify workforce needs that will be necessary to support clinical trials.
- Given the defined workforce, discuss the needs for career paths and career development opportunities.

SHERINE GABRIEL, *Session Chair*
William J. and Charles H. Mayo Professor of Medicine & Epidemiology Mayo Medical School
Co-Principal Investigator and Director of Education, Mayo Clinical Center for Translational Scientific Activities (CTSA)

1:15 p.m.   Presentation of Discussion Paper: *Developing a Robust Clinical Trials Workforce*

ROBERT CALIFF
Director, Duke Translational Medicine Institute
Professor of Medicine
Vice Chancellor for Clinical and Translational Research
Duke University Medical Center

ELAINE GALLIN
Principal
QE Philanthropic Advisors

MICHAEL LAUER
Director, Division of Cardiovascular Sciences
National Heart, Lung, and Blood Institute
National Institutes of Health

2:15 p.m.   **Panel Discussion with Speakers:** *Developing and*
              Sustaining a Clinical Trials Workforce
              Objectives:
              • List key skills, techniques, and areas of expertise needed
                by the workforce.
              • What are the benchmarks and metrics of success for an
                effective clinical trials workforce?
              • Propose and discuss the core competencies of a clinical
                trials workforce.

              SHERINE GABRIEL, *Panel Moderator*
              William J. and Charles H. Mayo Professor of Medicine &
              Epidemiology Mayo Medical School
              Co-Principal Investigator and Director of Education,
              Mayo Clinical Center for Translational Scientific
              Activities (CTSA)

              BRIGGS W. MORRISON
              Senior Vice President, Worldwide Medical Excellence
              Pfizer Inc.

              REBECCA JACKSON
              Professor and Associate Dean for Clinical Research
              Director and Principal Investigator,
              OSU Center for Clinical and Translational Science
              The Ohio State University

3:00 p.m.   BREAK

3:15 p.m.   **Keynote Address:** *Sustaining Institutional Support and*
              Patient Engagement in Clinical Trials: Models and Mes-
              sages from the NIH Clinical Center

              JOHN GALLIN
              Director
              National Institutes of Health Clinical Center

3:45 p.m.   **Discussion with Keynote Speaker, Panelists, and**
              Workshop Participants:
              • What are the needs for patient and broader public engage-
                ment in clinical trials?

- Discuss broad as well as disease-specific efforts to partner with patients in the development and conduct of clinical trials. How might these partnerships help create a national culture of clinical research in the United States?
- How can models and best practices from the NIH Clinical Center be adapted to the realities of other institutions and community systems to advance and promote the conduct of clinical trials in those systems?

JANET TOBIAS, *Moderator*
Co-founder and Partner, Ikana Health
Adjunct Assistant Professor,
Mount Sinai School of Medicine

ANNETINE GELIJNS
Professor of Health Policy
Co-Chair, Department of Health Evidence and Policy
Mount Sinai School of Medicine

HEATHER SNYDER
Senior Associate Director, Scientific Grants
Medical and Scientific Relations
Alzheimer's Association

4:30 p.m.   ADJOURN

Envisioning a Transformed Clinical Trials Enterprise in the United States: Establishing an Agenda for 2020

NOVEMBER 8, 2011

8:30 a.m.   Breakfast available

9:00 a.m.   Welcome and Introductions

JEFFREY DRAZEN, *Workshop Chair*
Editor-in-Chief
New England Journal of Medicine

SESSION III:
ALIGNING CULTURAL AND FINANCIAL INCENTIVES

Session Objective:
- Consider institutional needs to support clinical trials including addressing cultural issues and aligning financial incentives to support and sustain an efficient clinical trials enterprise.

ARTHUR H. RUBENSTEIN, *Session Chair*
Professor, Department of Medicine,
Division of Endocrinology
Raymond and Ruth Perelman School of Medicine
University of Pennsylvania

9:10 a.m.   Presentation of Discussion Paper: *Transforming the Economics of Clinical Trials*

JUDITH KRAMER
Associate Professor of Medicine,
Duke University Medical Center
Executive Director,
Clinical Trials Transformation Initiative (CTTI)

KEVIN SCHULMAN
Professor of Medicine and Business Administration
Duke University School of Medicine and
The Fuqua School of Business

9:50 a.m.   **Panel Discussion with Speakers:** *Aligning Cultural and Financial Incentives to Support Clinical Trials*
Objectives:
- Discuss incentives, reward structures, and business models impacting the conduct of clinical trials, and the key needs and challenges for advancing and improving upon these models.
- Consider regulatory, financial, and cultural changes that are needed to improve the environment for clinical trials.

ARTHUR H. RUBENSTEIN, *Panel Moderator*
Professor, Department of Medicine,
Division of Endocrinology
Raymond and Ruth Perelman School of Medicine
University of Pennsylvania

RICHARD RUDICK
Hazel Prior Hostetler Chair of Neurology,
Cleveland Clinic
Professor of Medicine,
Cleveland Clinic Lerner College of Medicine
Case Western Reserve University

CHRISTOPHER BEARDMORE
Chief Executive Officer
Translational Research Management

SCOTT STEELE
Director, Research Alliances
Adjunct Associate Professor,
Community and Preventive Medicine
University of Rochester

10:35 a.m.   BREAK

SESSION IV:
BUILDING AN INFRASTRUCTURE TO SUPPORT A TRANSFORMED CLINICAL TRIALS ENTERPRISE

Session Objectives:
- Set out an organizational framework for an infrastructure to conduct clinical trials.
- Discuss:
  — organizational frameworks for the infrastructure (i.e., network models or other approaches);
  — informatics needs;
  — regulatory reform or harmonization both within the United States and internationally.

CLYDE YANCY, *Session Chair*
Magerstadt Professor of Medicine
Chief, Division of Cardiology
Feinberg School of Medicine
Northwestern University

10:55 a.m.   Presentation of Discussion Paper: ***Developing a Clinical Trials Infrastructure***

> PETRA KAUFMANN
> Director, Office of Clinical Research
> National Institute of Neurological Disorders and Stroke
> National Institutes of Health

> PAUL EISENBERG
> Senior Vice President
> Global Regulatory Affairs and Safety
> Amgen Inc.

> JANET WOODCOCK
> Director, Center for Drug Evaluation and Research
> U.S. Food and Drug Administration

11:45 a.m.   **Panel Discussion with Speakers:** *Establishing an Infrastructure to Support a Transformed Clinical Trials Enterprise*
Objectives:
- Consider the types of trials that should be done in the United States and what the site/locus for the conduct of these trials should be within the infrastructure model proposed.
- What are the roles and responsibilities of the various participants and stakeholders in the proposed infrastructure of the clinical trials enterprise?

> CLYDE YANCY, *Panel Moderator*
> Magerstadt Professor of Medicine
> Chief, Division of Cardiology
> Feinberg School of Medicine
> Northwestern University

> LOUIS FIORE
> Principal Investigator, VA Cooperative Studies Program
> Director, VA Cooperative Studies Program Coordinating Center, Boston
> Department of Veterans Affairs

> MICHAEL KING JOLLY
> Senior Vice President
> Quintiles Innovation

KAREN MARGOLIS
Professor of Medicine,
University of Minnesota Medical School
Director of Clinical Research
HealthPartners Research Foundation

12:30 p.m. LUNCH

SESSION V:
DEVELOPING AN AGENDA FOR THE CREATION OF A TRANSFORMED CLINICAL TRIALS ENTERPRISE

Session Objectives:
- Define the key steps and responsible parties needed to achieve the elements of a transformed clinical trials enterprise discussed during the workshop.
- Consider the prioritization of transforming different elements of the clinical trials enterprise—what is feasible and most desirable?
- Consider any unintended consequences of transforming the clinical trials enterprise.
- Suggest a transformative path forward for decision makers and those implementing the work of clinical trials across the enterprise.

1:30 p.m. JEFFREY DRAZEN, *Session Chair*
Editor-in-Chief
New England Journal of Medicine

Presentation of Key Themes/Suggested Paths from Session Chairs

ALASTAIR J.J. WOOD, *Session I Chair*
Partner & Managing Director
Symphony Capital

SHERINE GABRIEL, *Session II Chair*
William J. and Charles H. Mayo Professor of Medicine
& Epidemiology Mayo Medical School
Co-Principal Investigator and Director of Education,
Mayo Clinical Center for Translational Scientific
Activities (CTSA)

ARTHUR H. RUBENSTEIN, *Session III Chair*
Professor, Department of Medicine,
Division of Endocrinology
Raymond and Ruth Perelman School of Medicine
University of Pennsylvania

CLYDE YANCY, *Session IV Chair*
Magerstadt Professor of Medicine
Chief, Division of Cardiology
Feinberg School of Medicine
Northwestern University

2:30 p.m.   ***Reflecting on Potential Paths Forward: Setting an Agenda
for a Transformed Clinical Trials Enterprise***

JEAN ROULEAU
Scientific Director
Institute for Circulatory and Respiratory Health
Canadian Institutes of Health Research (CIHR)

JEFFREY DRAZEN, *Panel Moderator*
Editor-in-Chief
New England Journal of Medicine

DOUGLAS CROPPER
President and Chief Executive Officer
Genesis Health System

LYNN ETHEREDGE
Co-Founder
Health Insurance Reform Project and Rapid Learning Project
George Washington University

RONALD KRALL
Associate Fellow
University of Pennsylvania, Center for Bioethics

JAMES DOROSHOW
Director, Division of Cancer Treatment and Diagnosis
National Cancer Institute, National Institutes of Health

4:30 p.m.   ADJOURN

Appendix B

Participant Biographies

Jeffrey M. Drazen, M.D. (*Workshop Chair*), was born in Missouri. He attended Tufts University, with a major in physics, and Harvard Medical School, and served his medical internship at Peter Bent Brigham Hospital in Boston. Thereafter, he joined the Pulmonary Divisions of the Harvard hospitals. He served as Chief of Pulmonary Medicine at the Beth Israel Hospital, Chief of the combined Pulmonary Divisions of the Beth Israel and Brigham and Women's Hospitals, and finally as the Chief of Pulmonary Medicine at Brigham and Women's Hospital. Through his research, he defined the role of novel endogenous chemical agents in asthma. This led to four new licensed pharmaceuticals for asthma with over 5 million people on treatment worldwide. In 2000, he assumed the post of Editor-in-Chief of the *New England Journal of Medicine*. During his tenure, the *Journal* has published major papers advancing the science of medicine, including the first descriptions of SARS and papers modifying the treatment of cancer, heart disease and lung disease. The *Journal*, which has over a million readers every week, has the highest impact factor of any journal publishing original research.

Christopher Beardmore began his career in regulatory affairs, influenced by leading human subject and animal subject protection committees at large academic institutions. While at the University of Maryland at Baltimore and the University of California at Los Angeles (UCLA) he reviewed and improved human subject protection systems, served as an advisor to streamline research processes, drafted policy and procedure manuals and developed training and education programs to improve systems. This included work with IRB members regarding review responsibilities and dealing extensively in issues related to ethical and regulatory training regarding GCP. Also while at UCLA, he represented all regulatory departments on an electronic research-networking database project designed to integrate regulatory affairs with budget and contract services. In September 2001, Mr. Beardmore relocated to Fort Detrick, Maryland, and worked with the U.S. Army Medical Research Institute of Infectious Disease to improve human subject activities. There he authored a position paper proposing innovative approaches to developing investigational biowarfare protective products. Over the years Mr. Beardmore has also consulted for numerous research hospitals, institutes, and IRBs including the West Los Angeles VA Medical Center, Friends Research Institute, and St. Johns Hospital/John Wayne Cancer Institute. All of these experiences led Mr. Beardmore to recognize a serious need to improve systems and permit ethical research to be conducted more efficiently. In 2004, he took on the role of Chief Operating Officer and Co-Founder of Premiere Oncology, a medical oncology research and treatment group operating in Santa Monica, California; San Diego, California; and Scottsdale, Arizona. Working with this group of practices until 2008, Mr. Beardmore established and streamlined the efforts of physicians, sites, and ancillary service providers and matched them with appropriate studies and sponsors to rapidly become one of the largest private Phase I groups in the United States. Mr. Beardmore found his vision for a community network of oncologists needed to be expanded beyond a single entity and left to form Translational Research Management (TRM) in 2009. TRM is dedicated to the creation of a community-focused clinical trial network, designed to bring innovative products to oncologists to potentially treat, ameliorate, or cure life-threatening or otherwise debilitating chronic disease. Currently TRM manages over 50 sites and is contracted with over 430 ancillary service providers who support those sites.

Robert Califf, M.D., graduated from Duke University, summa cum laude and Phi Beta Kappa, in 1973 and from Duke University Medical School in 1978, where he was selected for Alpha Omega Alpha. He performed his internship and residency at the University of California at San Francisco and his fellowship in cardiology at Duke University. He is board certified in internal medicine (1984) and cardiology (1986) and is a Master of the American College of Cardiology (2006). He is currently Vice Chancellor for Clinical Research, Director of the Duke Translational Medicine Institute (DTMI), and Professor of Medicine in the Division of Cardiology at the Duke University Medical Center in Durham, North Carolina. For 10 years he was the Founding Director of the Duke Clinical Research Institute (DCRI), the premier academic research organization in the world. He is the editor-in-chief of Elsevier's *American Heart Journal*, the oldest cardiovascular specialty journal. He has been author or co-author of more than 800 peer-reviewed journal articles and a contributing editor for theheart.org, an online information resource for academic and practicing cardiologists. He was recently acknowledged as one of the 10 most cited authors in the field of medicine by the Institute for Scientific Information (ISI). Dr. Califf led the DCRI for many of the best-known clinical trials in cardiovascular disease. With an annual budget of over $100 million, the DCRI has more than 1,000 employees and collaborates extensively with government agencies, the medical-products industry, and academic partners around the globe in all therapeutic areas. In cooperation with his colleagues from the Duke Databank for Cardiovascular Disease, Dr. Califf has written extensively about the clinical and economic outcomes of chronic heart disease. He is considered an international leader in the fields of health outcomes, quality of care, and medical economics. Dr. Califf's role as Director of the Duke Translational Medicine Institute, which is funded in part by an NIH CTSA, includes service as co-chairman of the Principal Investigators Steering Committee of the CTSA. Dr. Califf has served on the Cardiorenal Advisory Panel of the FDA and the Pharmaceutical Roundtable of the IOM. He served on the IOM committees that recommended Medicare coverage of clinical trials as well as the removal of ephedra from the market and on the IOM's Committee on Identifying and Preventing Medication Errors. He is currently a member of the IOM Forum on Drug Discovery, Development, and Translation and a subcommittee of the Science Board of FDA. He was the founding director of the coordinating center for the Centers for Education & Research on Therapeutics (CERTs), a public–private partnership among the Agency for Healthcare Research and Quality, FDA, academia, the medical-products industry, and consumer groups. This partnership focuses on research and education that will advance the best use of medical products. He is now the co-chairman of the CTTI, a public–private partnership focused on improving the clinical trials system.

Doug Cropper, M.H.A., is President and CEO of Genesis Health System (GHS) based in the Quad Cities area of Iowa and Illinois. GHS is a not-for-profit system offering a full continuum of health care services to a 10-county area. With an A1 Bond rating, GHS reported total operating revenue of $558 million in fiscal year 2010 and employs over 5,000 people. GHS has been the recipient of numerous awards and recognitions, including Thomson Reuters 50 Top Heart Hospitals, Thomson Reuters Top 50 Health Systems, 2010 J.D. Powers and Associates Distinguished Hospital for Providing "An Outstanding Patient Experience," a Top 100 IHS, 100

Most Wired Hospitals and Health Systems, Nursing Magnet designation, and the Consumer Choice Award from National Research Corporation. Mr. Cropper has more than 30 years of health care experience, starting out as a surgical orderly at St. Mark's Hospital in Salt Lake City, Utah. Prior to Genesis, he was Executive Vice President of Inova Health System and Administrator of the Inova Fairfax Hospital Campus in Falls Church, Virginia. Previous to his 5-year tenure at Inova, he served as Administrator of St. John's and St. Joseph's Hospitals and Vice President of HealthEast in St. Paul, Minnesota. Mr. Cropper graduated magna cum laude with a B.S. in history from the University of Utah (1984) and received a master's in Healthcare Administration from the University of Minnesota in 1988.

James H. Doroshow, M.D., FACP, has been the Director of the Division of Cancer Treatment and Diagnosis (DCTD), NCI, NIH, since 2004. He fosters collaboration with other NCI divisions and offices, as well as extramural scientists and clinicians, patient advocates, and professional cancer organizations. He leads the DCTD professional staff, who represent a wide array of scientific specialties, to integrate their insights and skills into a crossdisciplinary, scientifically driven, cooperative research endeavor to discover and develop better diagnostic and therapeutic interventions for cancer. Dr. Doroshow also oversees his own active laboratory program focusing on two lines of research: discovering the mechanisms that drive the anthracycline antibiotic cell death program and understanding the role of oxidative signals in the development and treatment of colon cancer. From 1983 to 2004, Dr. Doroshow was the Associate Director for Clinical Research at the City of Hope's (COH) Comprehensive Cancer Center in Duarte, California; the Chairman of the COH Department of Medical Oncology and Therapeutics Research; and the Leader of the COH Cancer Center's Clinical and Experimental Therapeutics Program. Through these roles, he oversaw solid tumor therapeutic research, supervised a staff of 75 involved in investigating novel targeted agents and other therapies, and directed a program of clinical research that supported more than 150 concurrently active clinical trials. While at COH, he founded an early therapeutics consortium of three NCI-designated cancer centers in California funded by both NCI's Phase I and II support grants. He was also the principal investigator for COH's membership in the Southwest Oncology Group (SWOG) and founding Chair of the SWOG Early Therapeutics Committee. From the time he received his first research grant in 1980, Dr. Doroshow was funded continuously by NCI and NIH until moving to NCI in 2004. He is the author of more than 300 full-length publications in the areas of the molecular and clinical pharmacology of the anthracycline antibiotics, the role of oxidant stress in signal transduction, and novel therapeutic approaches to breast, gastrointestinal, lung, and gynecologic cancer. Dr. Doroshow is a senior editor of *Clinical Cancer Research*. He is a member of the editorial boards of the *International Journal of Oncology, Technology in Cancer Research and Treatment,* and *Oncology*. He is also an associate editor for the widely used *Manual of Clinical Oncology* published by the International Union Against Cancer. Dr. Doroshow served from 1995 to 2001 as a member of the Subspecialty Board on Medical Oncology of the American Board of Internal Medicine, from 1999 to 2000 as Chair of NCI's Scientific Review Group-A Cancer Centers, and from 1990 to 1992 as Chair of the NIH Experimental Therapeutics II Study Section. He is currently a member of the FDA Oncologic Drugs Advisory Committee. Dr. Doroshow received his bachelor's degree, magna cum laude, from Harvard College in 1969 and his medical degree, Alpha Omega Alpha, from Harvard Medical School in 1973. After completing an internship and residency at Massachusetts General Hospital in Boston, he spent 3 years (1975-1978) at NCI as a clinical associate. He is board certified in internal medicine and medical oncology. Prior to joining COH in 1981, he held the position of Assistant Professor of Medicine in the Division of Medical Oncology at the University of Southern California School of Medicine in Los Angeles.

Paul R. Eisenberg, M.D., M.P.H., FACP, is the Senior Vice President of Global Regulatory Affairs and Safety at Amgen, effective February 2008. He was promoted after serving as Vice President of Global Regulatory Affairs and Safety since January 2007, and Vice President of Global Safety since December 2005. Prior to joining Amgen, Dr. Eisenberg was the Vice President of Lilly Global Product Safety. At Lilly he also led Clinical Development teams in Cardiovascular, Critical Care, and Inflammation Therapeutic Areas as Vice President–Internal Medicine and in discovery as Executive Director of Cardiovascular Research and Clinical Investigation. Dr. Eisenberg received his M.D. from New York Medical College and M.P.H. in Tropical Medicine from Tulane University School of Public Health. He was a Professor of Medicine at Washington University in St. Louis where his academic career, over 18 years, was focused on basic and clinical research in cardiovascular disease and thrombosis. This work led to over 100 publications in peer-reviewed journals and books. He has been involved in the discovery and development of numerous new molecular entities (NMEs) in both his academic and industry career. Dr. Eisenberg has led the development and registration of multiple NMEs in cardiovascular and critical care. In addition, he has extensive experience in global safety and risk management programs for drug development programs and postmarketing in multiple therapeutic classes.

Lynn M. Etheredge is an independent consultant on health care and social policy issues and heads the Rapid Learning Project at George Washington University. His career started at the White House Office of Management and Budget (OMB), where he was OMB's principal analyst for Medicare and Medicaid and led its staff work on national health insurance proposals. Mr. Etheredge headed OMB's professional health staff in the Carter and Reagan administrations. Later, he was a co-author of the Jackson Hole Group's proposals for health care reform. In 2007, he proposed the concept of the "rapid-learning health system" and is collaborating widely in developing this approach. Mr. Etheredge's recent publications include "Creating a High-Performance System for Comparative Effectiveness Research" and "Medicare's Future: Cancer Care." He serves on the editorial board of *Health Affairs*. He is author of more than 85 publications and is a graduate of Swarthmore College.

Gary L. Filerman, Ph.D., is President of the Atlas Health Foundation, an organization that addresses rural veteran's health services access issues and quality of care in corrections. He is adjunct professorial lecturer at the George Washington University School of Public Health and Health Services. He is also advisor to Joint Commission International, focusing on global health standards and relationships with international organizations and is an Open Society Institute faculty mentor. He formerly served at professor and chairman of the Department of Health Systems Administration at Georgetown University. Prior to joining Georgetown in 2000 he was for 2 years professor and interim chairman of the Department of Health Services and Policy at the George Washington University. Dr. Filerman joined the Georgetown faculty after a long career as the global leader in the development of management capacity and competency for health services. For 28 years he headed the Association of University Programs in Health Administration, a consortium of university, institute, and ministry programs in 30 countries. With the support of the W.K. Kellogg Foundation, Pew Trusts, the Robert Wood Johnson Foundation, the Commonwealth Fund, the World Health Organization (WHO), the U.S. Agency for International Development (USAID), and multinational corporations, his efforts focused upon the assessment of health system management needs, the design of university programs, and faculty and curriculum development and evaluation. He later served as vice president for international development of Planned Parenthood Federation of America, associate director of the Pew Commission on the Future of the Health Professions, senior health advisor at the Academy for Educational Development, consultant to the World Bank private health sector initiative, workforce leader for the World Bank Romania health sector reform, and headed planning for the 1997 Tashkent conference on NIS medical education reform. He has served as a consultant to ministries of health, universities, and health systems in 38 countries. Dr. Filerman has published widely on health care management development. He earned master's degrees in Latin American government and health services administration and his Ph.D. in health services from the University of Minnesota. He has been honored by the University of Leuven, the University of Puerto Rico, The Ohio State University, the University of Chicago, and with the Distinguished Contribution Award of the Regents of the University of Minnesota. He serves on several boards, including Volunteers of America. The endowed Filerman Prize is the highest recognition of leadership and scholarship in health systems administration education.

Louis Fiore, M.D., M.P.H., was born in Brooklyn, New York, and attended the State University of New York in Stony Brook (chemistry) and Upstate Medical Center in Syracuse (M.D.). He completed his residency and fellowships in hematology and oncology at the Boston VA and obtained an M.P.H. from the Harvard School of Public Health. Dr. Fiore has been an intramural researcher within the VA for 20 years. He was the Principal Investigator of the CHAMP Trial, a secondary prevention study of AMI that enrolled 5,000 subjects to either aspirin alone or in combination with warfarin. In 1996 he founded the Massachusetts Veterans Epidemiology Research and Information Center (MAVERIC), an epidemiology center within the VA Cooperative Studies Program. In 2002 the Center was expanded to include a clinical trials coordinating center. Since 2009 he has focused on bringing medical informatics expertise to the Program. His current interest lies in applying the disciplines of clinical trials, epidemiology, and informatics to integrate research into clinical care. To this end he has established the Point of Care Clinical Trials program in the VA.

Sherine E. Gabriel, M.D., M.Sc., is Professor of Medicine (Rheumatology) and Professor of Epidemiology, and the William J. and Charles H. Mayo Endowed Professor. She is currently Co-Principal Investigator and Director of Education, Center for Clinical and Translational Sciences, and Medical Director for Strategic Alliances and Business Development at Mayo Clinic. She is a Past President of the American College of Rheumatology. Dr. Gabriel's research, which is largely NIH-funded, has resulted in more than 350 peer-reviewed scientific publications addressing the risks, costs, determinants, and outcomes of the rheumatic diseases. She has received numerous research awards in recognition of these contributions. On January 21, 2011, Dr. Gabriel was appointed by the U.S. General Accountability Office to the Methodology Committee of PCORI and, soon after, was appointed as its first chair. PCORI was created by the U.S. Patient Protection and Affordable Care Act of 2010 as a nonprofit, nongovernmental organization to help patients, clinicians, purchasers, policy makers, and others make better-informed health decisions by carrying out research that provides high-quality, relevant evidence about interventions and strategies to prevent, diagnose, treat, and monitor health conditions. Dr. Gabriel earned a Doctor of Medicine degree, with distinction, from the University of Saskatchewan, Canada, completed internal medicine residency and rheumatology fellowship at Mayo Graduate School of Medicine and a master of science in clinical epidemiology from McMaster University. She is certified by the American Board of Internal Medicine in internal medicine and in rheumatology.

Elaine K. Gallin, Ph.D., is currently a partner at QE Philanthropic Advisors, a consulting firm established in 2010 that serves nonprofits specializing in biomedical research, science and math education, and international health. From 1999 through February 2010, Dr. Gallin served as the Doris Duke Charitable Foundation's (DDCF's) first Program Director for Medical Research. In that capacity, she led the creation and management of a portfolio of grant programs that committed more than $185 million to supporting clinical research. Dr. Gallin also designed and led DDCF's $65 million African Health Initiative. Launched in September 2007, this initiative supports large-scale health services delivery projects designed to provide integrated primary health care linked to rigorous operations and implementation research in several sub-Saharan African communities. Before joining DDCF, Dr. Gallin spent two decades working for the U.S. government, first as a research physiologist and then as research administrator where she last served as the Deputy Director of the Office of International Health Programs in the U.S. Department of Energy overseeing health research programs in countries of the former Soviet Union. During this period, she also spent a sabbatical year working in the Science Committee of the U.S. House of Representatives as a Congressional Science Fellow. Dr. Gallin has participated in numerous professional committees and review panels, including several for IOM and NIH. She was a founding member and the first Vice Chair of the Health Research Alliance (an alliance of not-for-profit, nongovernmental research funders). Dr. Gallin is currently a member of the Sickle Cell Disease Advisory Committee at the National Heart Lung and Blood Institute, the Forum on Drug Discovery, Development, and Translation at IOM, the Scientific Advisory Board for the Avon Foundation, and the President's Council of Cornell Women. Dr. Gallin received her B.S. from Cornell University and her Ph.D. from the City University of New York, and completed postdoctoral fellowships in physiology at Johns Hopkins University Medical School and Columbia University Medical School.

John I. Gallin, M.D., was appointed director of the NIH Clinical Center in 1994. The Clinical Center serves the clinical research needs of 17 NIH institutes and is the largest hospital in the world totally dedicated to clinical research. During his tenure, Dr. Gallin has overseen the design and construction of a new research hospital for the Clinical Center, the Mark O. Hatfield Clinical Research Center, which opened to patients in 2005; the establishment of a new curriculum for clinical research training now offered globally; and development of new information systems for biomedical translational and clinical research. While serving as Clinical Center director, Dr. Gallin has continued to be an active clinician and researcher. His primary research interest is in a rare hereditary immune disorder, chronic granulomatous disease (CGD). His laboratory described the genetic basis for several forms of CGD and has done pioneering research that has reduced life-threatening bacterial and fungal infections in CGD patients. A New York native, Dr. Gallin attended public school in New Rochelle, NY, graduated cum laude from Amherst College, and earned an M.D. degree at Cornell University Medical College. After a medical internship and residency at New York University's Bellevue Hospital Medical Center, he received postdoctoral training in basic and clinical research in infectious diseases at NIH from 1971 to 1974. He then went back to the New York University-Bellevue Medical Center as senior chief medical resident from 1974 to 1975 before returning to NIH. In 1985, Dr. Gallin began a 9-year period as scientific director for intramural research activities at the NIAID. Dr. Gallin was the founding chief of Laboratory of Host Defenses, NIAID, served as chief of the laboratory for 12 years, and continues as chief of the lab's clinical pathophysiology section. He has published more than 325 articles in scientific journals and has edited two textbooks: *Inflammation, Basic Principles and Clinical Correlates* (Lippincott, Williams, and Wilkins, 1999, now in its third edition) and *Principles and Practices of Clinical Research* (Academic Press, 2002, now in its second edition). Dr. Gallin is a member of the American Society for Clinical Investigation, the Association of American Physicians, and the IOM of the National Academy of Sciences, and he is a Master of the American College of Physicians.

Annetine C. Gelijns, Ph.D., is the Co-Chair of the Department of Health Evidence & Policy at Mount Sinai School of Medicine, New York, New York. Dr. Gelijns also holds the positions Professor of Health Policy, and Co-Director of the International Center for Health Outcomes and Innovation Research (InCHOIR) at Mount Sinai School of Medicine. Before coming to Mount Sinai in 2008, she was Professor of Public Health and Surgical Sciences in the Department of Surgery, College of Physicians and Surgeons, and the Division of Health Policy and Management of the Mailman School of Public Health, Columbia University, New York City. She was also a Division Chief in the Department of Surgery. Prior to her position at Columbia, she directed the Program on Technological Innovation in Medicine at the IOM, National Academy of Sciences. From 1983 to 1987, she worked for the Steering Committee on Future Health Scenarios and for the Health Council, the Netherlands. Dr. Gelijns has been a consultant to various national and international organizations, including WHO and the Organisation for Economic Co-operation and Development (OECD). Her research focuses on measurement of the long-term clinical outcomes and economic impact of clinical interventions, patient safety research, and the factors driving the development and diffusion of medical technology. She has special expertise in cardiovascular disease, particularly in the design, coordination, and analysis of multicenter trials. She is the PI or Co-PI of several Data Coordinating Centers for NHLBI-sponsored trials, including CT Surgery Clinical Trials Network, the REMATCH trial, and several newer generations of LVAD trials. Dr. Gelijns has published, in such journals as the *New England Journal of Medicine*, the *Journal of the American Medical Association*, and *Health Affairs*, on the methodology and conduct of complex surgical and device trials, the assessment of quality of life and economic analysis of clinical procedures, and volume-outcome studies, as well as policy studies on technological change.

Rebecca D. Jackson, M.D., is the Associate Dean for Clinical Research, Professor of Medicine and Director of the Center for Women's Health at The Ohio State University. She also serves as the founding Director of the OSU Center for Clinical and Translational Science and the Principal investigator of OSU's CTSA from NIH. Dr. Jackson received both her undergraduate and medical degree from The Ohio State University and her internship and residency training in internal medicine at Johns Hopkins Hospital. She returned to Ohio State in 1981 to complete her fellowship training in endocrinology and joined the faculty as an Assistant Professor of Endocrinology, Diabetes and Metabolism in 1983. Dr. Jackson has had a commitment to clinical and translational research throughout her academic career with a focus on examining and finding solutions to women's health issues, particularly osteoporosis and chronic musculoskeletal diseases associated with aging. Continuously federally funded since arriving at Ohio State, her individual and collaborative research efforts have resulted in peer-reviewed publications in the *Journal of the American Medical Association*, the *New England Journal of Medicine, Annals of Internal Medicine*, the *Journal of Bone and Mineral Research*, and other general medicine and subspecialty journals. She was lead author of the Women's Health Initiative analyses that showed that calcium plus vitamin D had a modest but nonsignificant effect on reducing hip fracture in postmenopausal women. Based upon its major scientific merit, this paper was selected for inclusion in the *Annual Bibliography of Significant Advances in Dietary Supplements Research* published by the Office of Dietary Supplements and NIH. Her recent efforts have focused on identifying genetic signatures and biomarkers for predicting risk for hip fracture, osteoarthritis, and cardiovascular disease. Her ultimate goal is to leverage this information to further elucidate the pathophyisology of these common complex diseases as well as to improve screening, prevention, and treatment. Dr. Jackson has served in leadership roles in both professional and scientific organizations including vice chair of the WHI Steering Committee from 2002 to 2010 and national co-chair of the CTSA Consortium in 2010 and she is currently a member of the Executive Committee of the NHLBI Exome Sequencing Project, the Executive Committee of the CTSA Consortium, the Board of Directors of the Clinical Research Forum, the NIH Advisory Board for Clinical Research, and secretary of the Society of Clinical and Translational Science. She has been the recipient of numerous awards and recognitions, including the NIH Physician Scientist Award and the Kellogg Foundation National Leadership Fellowship, and she is a member of Alpha Omega Alpha and a fellow of the American Association for the Advancement of Science. Dr. Jackson, who for more than a decade has been named one of "America's Best Doctors" by *U.S. News & World Report*, is also a member of the Ohio Women's Hall of Fame, has been recognized as a YWCA Woman of Achievement, and was named an American Medical Women's Association Legend.

Michael King Jolly, Pharm.D., is Senior Vice President of Quintiles Drug Development Innovation, where he leads drug development teams for partnered programs. Chief among his responsibilities are structuring and managing drug development collaborations with pharmaceutical companies. Dr. Jolly's pharmaceutical career began at Burroughs Wellcome Co. (BW) in 1983. While at BW, he served as Project Leader for over five new molecular entities in cardiovascular medicine and Brand Leader for LANOXIN brand digoxin for heart failure. Dr. Jolly first joined Quintiles in 1995 and led a strategic business unit that provided oversight of more than 40 cardiovascular product development programs ranging from Pre-IND to Phase IV. In 2000, he took a position at King Pharmaceuticals as Executive Vice President, where he formed a multidisciplinary research and development organization using a "virtual development model" in which outsourced partners performed all operations work, directed by a small core of functional experts. In early 2007, Dr. Jolly returned to Quintiles, joining NovaQuest. Dr. Jolly also teaches at Duke University Medical School and the School of Pharmacy at the University of North

Carolina (UNC) at Chapel Hill. Dr. Jolly received his undergraduate degree from UNC at Chapel Hill, and a Doctor of Pharmacy from the University of Texas at San Antonio. He subsequently completed a fellowship in clinical drug research and drug development from UNC at Chapel Hill and BW. Dr. Jolly is also a graduate of the Burroughs Wellcome Management Institute.

Petra Kaufmann, M.D., M.Sc., is the Director of NINDS Office of Clinical Research. Dr. Kaufmann is among the foremost experts in the design and management of clinical trials for neuromuscular disorders, including spinal muscular atrophy (SMA), amyotrophic lateral sclerosis (ALS), and mitochondrial diseases. Dr. Kaufmann leads the Institute's efforts to increase the effectiveness of clinical studies by addressing issues such as optimal trial design, ethical safe conduct of trials, and challenges in patient enrollment. Dr. Kaufmann has experience in all phases of clinical research, from conducting laboratory investigation and studies on disease mechanism to serving in key leadership positions on several major multicenter trials. Prior to her appointment at NINDS in 2009, Dr. Kaufmann was co-director of the SMA Clinical Research Center and an associate professor of neurology at Columbia University's Neurological Institute, where she had been a faculty member since 2000. She was also director of Columbia's clinical trials unit within the Pediatric Neuromuscular Clinical Research Network for SMA. Throughout her career, Dr. Kaufmann has implemented novel tools and techniques in clinical trials, including the development of web-based data management systems, telephone-administered neurological scales, imaging tests in ALS, and magnetic resonance spectroscopy to measure a biomarker in mitochondrial disorders.

Ronald Lee Krall, M.D., is Associate Fellow, University of Pennsylvania Center for Bioethics, and Former Chief Medical Officer for GlaxoSmithKline (retired). He is a member of the Executive Board of the Observational Medical Outcomes Partnership and of the Scientific Advisory Board of Kala Pharmaceuticals, and he consults for a number of health care companies. Dr. Krall holds a B.A. in mathematics from Swarthmore College and an M.D. from the University of Pittsburgh, and he completed his training in neurology and received a fellowship in clinical pharmacology at the University of Rochester. Over 25 years in the pharmaceutical industry, Dr. Krall worked for four companies (Lorex Pharmaceuticals, Abbott Laboratories, Zeneca/AstraZeneca, and GlaxoSmithKline), holding a variety of positions responsible for drug development, and safety of medicines. He concluded his career as Senior Vice President and Chief Medical Officer for GlaxoSmithKline. Over his career he has overseen in some capacity the development of over 20 medicines, including Ambien, Hytrin for benign prostatic hypertrophy, Depakote for migraine and bipolar disorder, Nolvadex, Arimidex and Faslodex for breast cancer, Seroquel, Accolate, Diprivan, Iressa, Tykerb, and Entereg.

Judith M. Kramer, M.D., M.S., has a broad background in both pharmacy and medicine, having worked in roles as practitioner, clinical researcher, scientific administrator, and policy advisor. Currently, she is Associate Professor of Medicine in the Division of General Internal Medicine at Duke University Medical Center, where she is involved full time in research-related activities. From 2000 to 2007, she was the principal investigator for Duke's Center for Education and Research on Therapeutics (CERTs), focused on cardiovascular disease. She has recently completed a term as Chairperson of FDA's Drug Safety and Risk Management (DSaRM) Advisory Committee. Since 2008 Dr. Kramer has been the Executive Director of the CTTI, a public–private partnership under FDA's Critical Path Program aimed at improving the quality and efficiency of clinical trials. Dr. Kramer received her B.S. and M.S. in pharmacy and M.D. from the University of North Carolina at Chapel Hill and is board certified in internal medicine. She did her residency in primary care internal medicine at Massachusetts General Hospital in Boston, and a senior residency in internal medicine at UNC Chapel Hill. After 5 years in practice of internal medicine in rural North Carolina, Dr. Kramer worked for 10 years at Burroughs Wellcome Co., where she became Vice President of Medical, directing U.S. clinical research. She continued in the merged GlaxoWellcome as International Director of Cardiovascular/Critical Care Clinical Research before leaving to work at Duke in 1996. At Duke she served as Chief Medical Officer of the Duke Clinical Research Institute from 1997 to 2006, and regulatory consultant to the Duke Translational Medicine Institute from 2006 to 2008. From 1999 to 2001, Dr. Kramer also served as the Founding Director of the Masters Program in Clinical Research at Campbell University, in Research Triangle Park, North Carolina. Dr. Kramer's research interests have focused on finding safe and effective cardiovascular therapies, ensuring persistent use of life-saving medications, and evaluating how clinical trials are conducted.

Michael S. Lauer, M.D., has served as Director of the Division of Cardiovascular Sciences at the NHLBI since October 14, 2009. Dr. Lauer is a cardiologist and clinical epidemiologist noted for his work on diagnostic testing, clinical manifestations of autonomic nervous system dysfunction, and clinical comparative effectiveness. Dr. Lauer received a B.S. in biology from the Rensselaer Polytechnic Institute and an M.D. from Albany Medical College; he also participated in the Program in Clinical Effectiveness at the Harvard School of Public Health. He received postgraduate training at Massachusetts General Hospital, Boston's Beth Israel Hospital, and the Framingham Heart Study. Prior to coming to NIH, Dr. Lauer was a professor of medicine, epidemiology, and biostatistics at the Cleveland Clinic Lerner College of Medicine of Case Western Reserve University and a Contributing Editor for the *Journal of the American Medical Association*. He is an elected member of the American Society of Clinical Investigation and won the Ancel Keys Award of the American Heart Association in 2008. In 2010 he won the NIH Equal Employment Opportunity (EEO) Award of the Year.

Bryan R. Luce, Ph.D., M.B.A., is Senior Vice President, Science Policy for United BioSource Corporation (UBC). Dr. Luce founded MEDTAP® International (now part of UBC), serving as its Chairman, President, and CEO until 2002. Previously, he held positions as Director of Battelle's Centers for Public Health Research and Evaluation, Director of the Office of Research and Demonstrations, CMS, and Senior Analyst, Office of Technology Assessment (OTA) of the U.S. Congress. Dr. Luce is a consultant to numerous government agencies as well as pharmaceutical and device firms worldwide, a member or chair of socioeconomic and public health policy advisory boards for several leading pharmaceutical companies, and recently was a member of the Medicare Evidence Development & Coverage Advisory Committee (MedCAC). He is a Senior Scholar with the Department of Health Policy, Jefferson Medical College, and has authored more than 90 scientific publications, including three textbooks on technology assessment, health policy, and cost-effectiveness analysis. In 2008, Dr. Luce founded the Pragmatic Approaches to Comparative Effectiveness (PACE) Initiative, whose mission is to explore novel analytical efficiency comparative effectiveness trial methods. Previously, he founded the Bayesian Initiative in Health Economics and Outcomes Research. He is a Past President of the International Society for Pharmacoeconomics and Outcomes Research (ISPOR) and, in 2008, received the Society's Avedis Donabedian Outcomes Research Lifetime Achievement Award. A former Special Forces Officer, Dr. Luce holds the rank of Lieutenant Colonel (Retired), Medical Service Corps, U.S. Army Reserves. His undergraduate and master's training were at the Universities of Vermont and Massachusetts at Amherst. He received his doctorate from the School of Public Health at the University of California at Los Angeles (UCLA).

Karen L. Margolis, M.D., M.P.H., is the Director of Clinical Research and a Senior Investigator at HealthPartners Research Foundation in Minneapolis, Minnesota. She is a board-certified internist and primary care physician with HealthPartners Medical Group. Dr. Margolis is a Professor of Medicine at the University of Minnesota Medical School, with an adjunct appointment in the School of Public Health's Division of Epidemiology and Community Health. She is a standing member of the Clinical Trials Review Committee for NHLBI. Dr. Margolis received her bachelor of science from the University of Michigan in 1979, her medical degree from the University of Michigan Medical School in 1983, and her Master of Public Health in Epidemiology from the University of Minnesota School of Public Health in 1992. Her research interests are in the areas of women's health, prevention of cardiovascular disease, and the epidemiology and treatment of hypertension and diabetes. She is a member of Phi Beta Kappa, Alpha Omega Alpha, the American College of Physicians, the Society of General Internal Medicine, the American Heart Association, the American Diabetes Association, and the American Society of Hypertension. Before she took her current position at HealthPartners, she was a faculty physician in the Department of Medicine at Hennepin County Medical Center in Minneapolis and Associate Medical Director of the Berman Center for Clinical Research. In 2003, Dr. Margolis spent a year as a guest researcher in the Department of Medical Epidemiology and Biostatistics at the Karolinska Institute in Stockholm, Sweden. She has served in leadership positions in many large multicenter, federally funded initiatives and trials, including the Antihypertensive and Lipid-Lowering Treatment to Prevent Heart Attack Trial (ALLHAT), the Women's Health Initiative, the Action to Control Cardiovascular Risks in Diabetes (ACCORD), and the ongoing Aspirin in Reducing Events in the Elderly (ASPREE) study. Dr. Margolis also leads and participates in investigator-initiated and industry-funded clinical trials, and is the site Principal Investigator for the NHLBI-funded Cardiovascular Research Network.

Briggs W. Morrison, M.D., is Senior Vice President and Head of Worldwide Medical Excellence working with teams across Business Units, Research and Development and Pfizer Medical to establish global systems, processes, and metrics to advance and evaluate clinical trials quality and compliance with GCPs and simultaneously improve cycle times. He was formerly Senior Vice President of the Primary Care Medicines Development Group and the Head of Clinical Development in the Global Research and Development Division of Pfizer Inc., leading all Clinical Development (Phase I to III) activities for Pfizer, overseeing all the Development Therapeutic Areas as well as Clinical Operations. Prior to joining Pfizer, Dr. Morrison held various positions of increasing responsibility in Clinical Development at Merck & Co., Inc. He received a B.S. in biology from Georgetown University in 1981 and earned his M.D. from the University of Connecticut in 1985. He completed his internship and residency in internal medicine in 1988 at the Massachusetts General Hospital, completed his Fellowship in Medical Oncology in 1991 at the Dana Farber Cancer Institute, and completed a postdoctoral fellowship in molecular oncology in 1994 at the Harvard Medical School/Howard Hughes Medical Institute under the guidance of Dr. Philip Leder.

Richard K. Murray, M.D., FACP, joined Merck & Co., Inc. in November 1994, where he was a founding member of the Regional Medical Director Program. Over the subsequent 17 years, he assumed increasing responsibility within U.S. Human Health Medical and Scientific Affairs, including head of U.S. Academic and Professional Affairs, and he was promoted to Vice President, External Medical and Scientific Affairs, in August of 2007. He became Head of the Global Center for Scientific Affairs in May 2010, including responsibility for the Merck Investigator-Initiated Studies Program. Dr. Murray, a native Washingtonian, graduated from Clark University (Worcester, Massachusetts) with an A.B. in psychology and an M.A. in chemistry. He graduated from Howard University College of Medicine (Washington, DC) and subsequently was an intern, medical resident, Chief Medical Resident, and Pulmonary and Critical Care Fellow at the University of Pennsylvania in Philadelphia. Prior to joining Merck, Dr. Murray was assistant professor of medicine at the University of Pennsylvania, where he was an investigator in the area of reactive airways disease, smooth muscle function, and calcium signaling. He was also Co-Director of the Adult Asthma Program at the Hospital of the University of Pennsylvania. Dr. Murray is board certified in internal medicine and pulmonary diseases. He is a Fellow of the American College of Physicians, a Fellow of the American College of Chest Physicians, and a Fellow of the College of Physicians of Philadelphia. He serves on the boards of directors for the Merck Childhood Asthma Network and the Southeast Pennsylvania Chapter of the American Heart Association. Dr. Murray has previously represented Merck at the IOM Clinical Research Roundtable and the Roundtable on Health Disparities.

Richard Platt, M.D., M.Sc., is a professor and chair of the Department of Population Medicine at Harvard Medical School and Executive Director of the Harvard Pilgrim Health Care Institute. He is principal investigator of the AHRQ HMORN DEcIDE Center, a CDC Prevention Epicenter, and a CDC Center of Excellence in Public Health Informatics. He also leads the FDA's Mini-Sentinel program and contracts with FDA's Center for Drug Evaluation and Research (CDER) and Center for Biologics Evaluation and Research (CBER) to conduct postmarketing studies of drugs' and biologics' safety and effectiveness. He chaired FDA's Drug Safety and Risk Management Advisory Committee, is a member of the Association of American Medical Colleges' Advisory Panel on Research, and the IOM

Roundtable on Value & Science-Driven Health Care. Dr. Platt was co-chair of the Board of Scientific Counselors of CDC's Center for Infectious Diseases. Additionally, he has chaired the NIH study section Epidemiology and Disease Control 2, and the CDC Office of Health Care Partnerships steering committee.

Ihor W. Rak, M.D., was born in New York City, graduated from The City College of New York, and earned his medical degree at the College of Physicians and Surgeons at Columbia University, New York City. He completed his internship, residency, and fellowship at the Hospital of the University of Pennsylvania and the Children's Hospital of Philadelphia. He has earned several medical board certifications (pediatrics, neurology, pediatric neurology, and clinical neurophysiology). After serving in the U.S. Air Force as Chief of Pediatric Neurology and Neurology Services in the U.S. Air Force Medical Corps, Wright-Patterson Air Force Base, Ohio, Dr. Rak was an assistant professor of neurology and research associate at the University of Virginia, Charlottesville, Virginia. Dr. Rak was Founder and Medical Director of the Epilepsy Center and Co-Director of the Sleep Disorders Center at Sacred Heart Hospital, Allentown, Pennsylvania. As Principal Investigator he continued his clinical research activities, contributing to many investigational antiepileptic drugs. Since joining AstraZeneca Global Clinical Research in 1996, he has provided medical and project team leadership for a number of clinical projects, including SEROQUEL. As Global Product Director for Emerging Neuroscience, he successfully led the global neurologic, psychiatric, and overactive bladder early development projects. In 2005 Dr. Rak was appointed Vice President, Global Clinical Development for the Neuroscience Therapy Area. In his current role, he oversees the development and delivery of the clinical contributions for both emerging products and established brands in the Global Neuroscience Therapy Area. Dr. Rak attended executive development programs at the University of Pennsylvania's Wharton School of Business and R&D Executive Leadership Program at Harvard Business School. He has held numerous leadership roles, including President and Chairman of the Board of Trustees with the American Academy of Pharmaceutical Physicians (AAPP, now APPI, the Academy of Pharmaceutical Physicians and Investigators) and Vice President of Strategic Planning the National Alliance for the Mentally Ill (NAMI), Delaware Chapter.

Jean L. Rouleau, M.D., is the Scientific Director of the Institute of Circulatory and Respiratory Health of the Canadian Institutes of Health and Research (CIHR). Dr. Rouleau was Dean of the University of Montreal's Faculty of Medicine from 2003 to 2010. He practices cardiology at the Montreal Heart Institute. He has also served as a member of the CIHR

Governing Council from 2005 to 2010. A respected cardiologist and world-famous researcher, Dr. Rouleau previously taught at the University of Toronto and served as Director of the Cardiac Program and the Cardiology departments at Toronto's University Health Network (UHN) and at Mount Sinai Hospital from 1999 to 2003. With experience in many university hospitals, Dr. Rouleau possesses a vast understanding of the worlds of teaching, research, and care settings. He earned his M.D. degree from the University of Ottawa and completed his clinical training at McGill University followed by postdoctoral research in San Francisco. Dr. Rouleau has published over 355 scientific articles in journals such as the *American Journal of Medicine*, the *American Journal of Cardiology*, the *Canadian Medical Association Journal*, *Lancet*, and the *New England Journal of Medicine*. He has been awarded the Canadian Centennial Medal, the Exceptional Merit Award given by the Fonds de la Recherche en Santé du Québec (FRSQ), the Canadian Henry Friesen Award, and the Canadian Cardiovascular Society's Career Research Achievement Award.

Arthur H. Rubenstein, M.B.B.Ch., is Professor, Department of Medicine, Division of Endocrinology at the Raymond and Ruth Perelman School of Medicine at the University of Pennsylvania. Previously, Dr. Rubenstein was the Executive Vice President of the University of Pennsylvania for the Health System and Dean of the Raymond and Ruth Perelman School of Medicine from September 2001 to July 2011. Together, these entities make up Penn Medicine, a $3.6 billion enterprise dedicated to the related missions of medical education, biomedical research, and excellence in patient care. Founded in 1765, Penn's Perelman School of Medicine received over $397.4 million in NIH research funds in fiscal year 2010. With 1,823 full-time faculty and nearly 3,000 students, trainees, residents, and fellows, the school is recognized worldwide for its superior education and training of the next generation of physician-scientists and leaders of academic medicine. The University of Pennsylvania Health System (UPHS) includes its flagship hospital, the Hospital of the University of Pennsylvania (HUP); Pennsylvania Hospital, the nation's first hospital; Penn Presbyterian Medical Center; and Penn Medicine at Rittenhouse. In addition, it encompasses a primary care provider network, a faculty practice plan, home care, hospice, and nursing home and three multispecialty satellite facilities. Before joining Penn, Dr. Rubenstein served for four years as Dean of Mount Sinai School of Medicine and Gustave L. Levy Distinguished Professor. Earlier, he was the Lowell T. Coggeshall Distinguished Service Professor of Medical Sciences and Chairman of the Department of Medicine at the University of Chicago Pritzker School of Medicine. Dr. Rubenstein is an internationally prominent endocrinologist recognized for clinical expertise and groundbreaking research in diabetes. Well known for his inspired teaching, Dr. Rubenstein has served in numerous professional leadership positions during his career. These include President of the Association of Professors of Medicine, President of the Association of American Physicians, President of the Central Society for Clinical Research, Chairman of the American Board of Internal Medicine, Chairman of the Board of the Association of Academic Health Centers, and Chair of the National Diabetes Advisory Board. He has been a member of a study section and of the Advisory Council of the National Institute of Diabetes and Digestive and Kidney Diseases. Author of more than 350 publications, Dr. Rubenstein has held editorial advisory positions with several respected journals, including service on the editorial boards of the *Annals of Internal Medicine*, the *Journal of Diabetes and Its Complications*, *Medicine*, and *Clinical Trials Advisor*. He was also a consulting editor to the *Journal of Clinical Investigation*. Dr. Rubenstein is the recipient of many awards and prizes, including the highest honor from the Association of Professors of Medicine, the Robert H. Williams Distinguished Chair of Medicine Award. Among his other honors are the John Phillips Memorial Award from the American College of Physicians; the Banting Medal from the American Diabetes Association; and the David Rumbough Scientific Award from the Juvenile Diabetes Association. In 2009, Dr. Rubenstein was awarded the prestigious Abraham Flexner Award for Distinguished Service to Medical Education from the Association of American Medical Colleges. Born in South Africa, Dr. Rubenstein received his medical degree from the University of the Witwatersrand in Johannesburg. In 2001, he was honored by his alma mater when an honorary degree, Doctor of Science in Medicine, was conferred upon him. He is a Fellow of the College of Medicine of South Africa and of the Royal College of Physicians of London; a Master of the American College of Physicians; American Academy of Arts and Sciences; and a member of the IOM of the National Academy of Sciences.

Richard A. Rudick, M.D., Professor of Medicine, Cleveland Clinic Lerner College of Medicine Hazel Prior Hostetler Chair of Neurology, Cleveland Clinic Director, Mellen Center for Multiple Sclerosis Treatment and Research, Cleveland Clinic Vice Chairman, Research and Development in the Neurological Institute, Cleveland Clinic. Dr. Rudick graduated from Case Western Reserve University School of Medicine in 1975. Following internship and residency in medicine at the University of Connecticut, Dr. Rudick trained in neurology at the University of Rochester. During a postdoctoral research fellowship in the Center for Brain Research at the University of Rochester, studies focused on neurologic consequences of immune complex disease in animal systems and immunologic abnormalities in multiple sclerosis (MS) patients. Dr. Rudick's subsequent studies on cerebrospinal fluid in MS were supported by an NIH clinical investigator career development award. In 1987, Dr. Rudick became Director of the Mellen Center. He has played key roles in several MS clinical trials, including pivotal registration trials of IFNβ-1a (Avonex) and natalizumab (Tysabri) for relapsing remitting MS. He continues studies on immunologic changes in MS patients, has led development of new clinical and imaging measures for MS trials, and maintains a consultative clinical practice at the Mellen Center. Dr. Rudick has maintained continuous competitive grant funding from NIH and National Multiple Sclerosis Society for over 25 years. In addition to being Director of the Mellen Center, Dr. Rudick is Vice Chairman of Research and Development in the Neurological Institute and Co–Principal Investigator of a citywide Clinical and Translational Science Collaborative.

Kevin A. Schulman, M.D., M.B.A., is a professor of medicine and the Gregory Mario and Jeremy Mario Professor of Business Administration at Duke University. He is an associate director of the Duke Clinical Research Institute at the Duke University School of Medicine. At Duke's Fuqua School of Business, he serves as director of the Health Sector Management Program, the Master of Management in Clinical Informatics, and the Center for the Study of Health Management. His other university affiliations include the Trent Center for Bioethics, Humanities and History of Medicine; the Duke Translational Research Institute Pilot Project Advisory Committee; and the Duke Global Health Institute. Dr. Schulman is a distinguished researcher who has received more than $34 million in research grants. His research interests include health services research and policy, including access to care and the impact of reimbursement and regulatory policies on clinical practice; health economics and economic evaluation in clinical research; and medical decision making, especially in patients with life-threatening conditions. He regularly teaches courses in biotechnology, health policy, and health IT strategy. Dr. Schulman has published more than 350 papers and book chapters; his peer-reviewed articles have appeared in the *New England Journal of Medicine*, the *Journal of the American Medical Association*, and *Annals of Internal Medicine*. He is a member of the editorial/advisory boards of the *American Journal of Medicine*, the *American Heart Journal*, *Health Services Research*, and *Value in Health*. A recipient of numerous awards, Dr. Schulman is a fellow of the American College of Physicians and an elected member of the American Society for Clinical Investigation. He has served as session chair and panelist at dozens of medical and health care conferences. Dr. Schulman has also served on numerous grant review committees for the NIH, the Robert Wood Johnson Foundation, and other bodies. He is a member of the advisory board for the Centre for Healthcare Policy and Management at the China Europe International Business School. In 2010–2011, he was a mentor for the Commonwealth Fund's Harkness Fellowships in Health Care Policy and Practice. He is a voting member of the Medicare Evidence Development and Coverage Advisory Committee. Dr. Schulman received his M.D. from the New York University School of Medicine and his M.B.A., with a concentration in health care management, from the Wharton School of the University of Pennsylvania. He completed a residency in internal medicine at the Hospital of the University of Pennsylvania and is board certified in internal medicine.

Heather M. Snyder, Ph.D., assists with oversight of the Alzheimer's Association International Research Grant Program, the world's largest nonprofit initiative to advance Alzheimer's research. Since 1982, the Association has committed $292 million to more than 2,000 best-of-field investigators worldwide. In addition to assisting with smooth review of proposals and distribution of awards to successful applicants, Dr. Snyder assumes primary responsibility for metrics and qualitative assessments to enhance the program's effectiveness and impact, and for communicating program results to a wide range of audiences. After earning an undergraduate degree in biology and religious studies at the University of Virginia, Dr. Snyder moved on to graduate and postgraduate studies in Chicago, completing her Ph.D. at Loyola University Chicago Stritch School of Medicine and a postdoctoral fellowship at Children's Memorial Research Center of Northwestern University.

Scott J. Steele, Ph.D., M.A., serves as the Director of Research Alliances at the University of Rochester. In this role he fosters strategic research partnerships between the University's research community and industry, government agencies and laboratories, and other academic institutions. He is actively involved with the University of Rochester Clinical and Translational Science Institute, serving as the Director of the Public–Private–Partnerships Key Function. Additionally, he holds an adjunct appointment in the Department of Community and Preventive Medicine. Prior to joining the University of Rochester, Dr. Steele served in the White House Office of Science and Technology Policy (OSTP), initially as a policy analyst and later designated as the Executive Director of the President's Council of Advisors on Science and Technology (PCAST). Dr. Steele coordinated PCAST studies addressing issues in personalized medicine, nanotechnology, energy technologies, and approaches to enhance university–private sector research partnerships. Previously, Dr. Steele served as a senior policy specialist and intelligence analyst at the Federal Bureau of Investigation (FBI), within the FBI's Weapons of Mass Destruction program. Dr. Steele received his B.S. with honors in biology from

Union College in Schenectady, New York. Following this, he performed research at the General Electric Center for Research and Development and was a fellow at NIH in Bethesda, Maryland. Dr. Steele completed his M.A. and Ph.D. in molecular biology at Princeton University.

Janet Tobias is a technology/media executive specializing in health care, and an Emmy Award–winning director/producer/writer. Ms. Tobias started her career at CBS' *60 Minutes* as Diane Sawyer's associate producer. At *60 Minutes* she distinguished herself working on a wide range of domestic and international stories including a portrait of the Yakuza, the Japanese organized crime syndicate, and investigations into the lack of regulation in infertility treatment and the abuse of boys in a Guatemalan orphanage. Ms. Tobias moved with Ms. Sawyer to ABC News to launch *Prime Time Live*. At ABC she produced and directed both domestic and international stories ranging from a case study of organ donation to a portrait of the Kuwaiti royal family after the first Gulf War. After a short stint away from the networks to write a feature film screenplay, Ms. Tobias returned to NBC and moved into management at *Dateline NBC*. As a national producer at *Dateline NBC*, she supervised pieces on medical ethics and the home health care industry. She also continued to produce and direct her own stories, ranging from a historical look back at Soviet misinformation campaigns to an investigation into oil development in the Ecuadoran rainforest. Ms. Tobias left NBC News to become an Executive Producer at VNI (which became *New York Times* Television). There she supervised the production of a foreign news show and reporting on a variety of foreign stories including an award-winning piece on rape as a war crime in Rwanda that appeared on *Nightline*. Ms. Tobias then returned to ABC News to head up editorial activities at its newly created Law and Justice Unit where she reported, directed, and supervised legal and criminal justice stories for all ABC news programs: *Nightline, 20/20, World News Tonight*, and *Good Morning America*. In 1998 Ms. Tobias began working as an executive with PBS, where she developed and produced programming not only for PBS but also joint projects with ABC and Discovery. She continued her directing and writing career, winning two American Bar Association silver gavels for a 4-hour *Frontline/Nightline* project on the juvenile justice system in California. In 2001, she launched *Life 360*, a weekly PBS series hosted by Michel Martin that combined documentary pieces with dramatic and comic monologues. *Life 360* launched just after 9/11 to laudatory reviews and won an Emmy in its first season. It was also one of two programs picked to pilot interactive television at PBS. In 2001, Ms. Tobias founded her own television/film production company, Sierra/Tango Productions. Sierra/Tango has produced over a dozen documentaries on social issues ranging from medical ethics to the life of teenagers in America. Currently, Ms. Tobias is directing a film for worldwide theatrical release, and television broadcast, on the longest ever recorded uninterrupted survival underground in a cave. In addition to her National Emmy and American Bar Association awards, other awards include two Cine Golden Eagles, the George Foster Peabody Award, two Casey medals for meritorious journalism, a National Headliner Award, a Sigma Delta Chi Award, and honorable mention Robert F. Kennedy Journalism and Overseas Press Awards. Ms. Tobias is a member of the Writers Guild of America. In 2002, Ms. Tobias moved into the technology world full time when she joined Sawyer Media Systems, a Sequoia Capital backed creator of video technology for the web. Ms. Tobias was a member of the executive committee at Sawyer Media Systems, where she supervised the web design and video teams. Cisco Systems bought the video portal Sawyer developed and incorporated it into their technical offerings. In 2004, Ms. Tobias was one of the founding partners of Ikana Media, now Ikana Health. In 2009, Ms. Tobias became the CEO of Ikana Health, which focuses on the mobile web, social media, and video as it relates to health care information and outcomes. Clients include AARP, Babycenter. com, Johnson & Johnson, St. Luke's Roosevelt Hospital, Mount Sinai School of Medicine, Cisco Systems, Time Inc., and WGBH. A graduate of Yale University, Ms. Tobias served from January to September 2009 as a senior fellow at the University of British Columbia, Sauder School of Business Centre for Sustainability and Social Innovation. In 2009, she was appointed to the Forum on Drug Discovery, Development, and Translation of the IOM, National Academy of Sciences. In 2010, Ms. Tobias became an adjunct assistant professor of Medicine in the Department of Health Evidence and Policy at Mount Sinai School of Medicine.

Neil J. Weissman, M.D., FACC, is President of MedStar Health Research Institute, Professor of Medicine at Georgetown University School of Medicine, and he directs the Cardiovascular Core Laboratories at Washington Hospital Center in Washington, DC. Dr. Weissman's research interests include valvular heart disease, left ventricular remodeling, and intravascular imaging. His ultrasound core laboratory has served as a site for over 150 multicenter trials, including multiple studies on pharmacologic effects of valvular and ventricular function, prosthetic valve assessments, and intracoronary therapies. Additionally, Dr. Weissman has served as principal investigator (PI) for numerous national and international multicenter trials; he recently was the national PI on a series of cardiac safety studies with over 8,000 participants. Dr. Weissman has published hundreds of abstracts and original reports in such well-regarded journals as the *New England Journal of Medicine*, the *Journal of the American Medical Association*, *Annals of Internal Medicine*, the *American Journal of Cardiology*, the *American Heart Journal*, and the *Journal of the American College of Cardiology*. He also has written several review articles and book chapters and wrote a textbook on cardiac imaging. Dr. Weissman received his medical degree from Cornell University Medical College in New York City. He then completed his internship, residency, and chief residency in internal medicine at the New York Hospital in New York City. He followed his residency training with a clinical and research fellowship in cardiology and a fellowship in cardiac ultrasound at Massachusetts General Hospital in Boston, Massachusetts. Prior to moving to the Washington Hospital Center, he was the director of the clinical echo lab at Georgetown University. Dr. Weissman is internationally recognized as an expert in cardiac ultrasound and served on several national organizations, including Chair of the Guidelines and Standards, Board of Directors and Executive Committee of the American Society of Echocardiography, Chair of the Program Committee for Imaging for the American College of Cardiology, and Chair of the Scientific Sessions for the American Society of Echocardiography. Dr. Weissman is often an invited expert on FDA Advisory Committee and NIH commissions.

Alastair J. J. Wood, M.D., was Professor of Medicine and Pharmacology, Assistant Vice Chancellor and Associate Dean at Vanderbilt Medical School before being appointed Emeritus Professor of Medicine and Emeritus Professor of Pharmacology in 2006. His current academic appointments are Professor of Medicine and Professor of Pharmacology at Weill Cornell Medical College, New York. He is a Partner at Symphony Capital LLC, a New York–based Private Equity Company. Dr. Wood is a member of the National Academy of Sciences IOM, the American Association of Physicians (AAP), the American Society for Clinical Investigation (ASCI), Honorary Fellow, American Gynecological and Obstetrical Society (AGOS), and Fellow of the American College of Physicians. Dr. Wood served on the *New England Journal of Medicine* Editorial Board and was the *NEJM Drug Therapy* Editor for many years. He authored the chapter in Harrison's *Principles of Internal Medicine on Adverse Drug Reactions* from the 9th through the 15th edition. He was the chairman of the FDA's Nonprescription Drugs Advisory Committee until 2006, and chaired the 2005 FDA Advisory Committee on Cox-2 inhibitors. He previously served as a member of the Cardiovascular and Renal Advisory Committee of FDA and the FDA's Nonprescription Drugs Advisory Committee. His research interests have been focused on understanding the mechanisms for interindividual variability in drug response and toxicity. His research has resulted in over 300 articles, reviews, and editorials.

Janet Woodcock, M.D., is the Director of the Center for Drug Evaluation and Research (CDER) at FDA. She also served as CDER Director from 1994 to 2005. Dr. Woodcock has held various positions within the Office of the Commissioner, FDA, from October 2003 to April 1, 2008. Prior to her 2008 reappointment to CDER, she served as Deputy Commissioner for Operations and Chief Operating Officer, where she was responsible for overseeing agency operations and crosscutting regulatory and scientific processes. She previously served in other positions at FDA, including Director, Office of Therapeutics Research and Review, and Acting Deputy Director, Center for Biologics Evaluation and Research. Dr. Woodcock received her M.D. from Northwestern Medical School and completed further training and held teaching appointments at the Pennsylvania State University and the University of California, San Francisco. She joined FDA in 1986.

Clyde W. Yancy, M.D., M.Sc., FACC, FAHA, MACP, is the newly appointed Chief of Cardiology at Northwestern University, Feinberg School of Medicine, and Associate Director of the Bluhm Cardiovascular Institute at Northwestern Memorial Hospital. He holds the Magerstadt Endowed Professor of Medicine Chair. Formerly he was the Medical Director, Baylor Heart and Vascular Institute at Baylor University Medical Center in Dallas, Texas, and Chief of Cardiothoracic Transplantation at Baylor University Medical Center, Dallas, Texas. He is board certified in internal medicine with a subspecialty in cardiovascular disease. He is a Fellow of the American College of Cardiology, a Fellow of the American Heart Association (AHA), and a Master of the American College of Physicians. He is also a member of the International Society of Heart and Lung Transplantation (ISHLT), the American Society of Hypertension (ASH), the Heart Failure Society of America (HFSA), and the Association of Black Cardiologists (ABC). He has previously served on the Executive Council of the HFSA, is past chair of the Education Committee of the HFSA, and past chair the Council of Clinical Cardiology's Heart Failure and Transplantation Sub-Committee of the AHA. Dr. Yancy has served two terms on the national Board of Directors for the AHA and was recognized as the AHA National Physician of the Year in 2003. He sits on the ACC/AHA Guideline Writing Committee for chronic heart failure and is a member of the ACC Guideline Taskforce which oversees all ACC/AHA guidelines. In 2009–2010, he served as President of the American Heart Association.

Peter Paul Yu, M.D., is in clinical practice at the Palo Alto Medical Foundation (PAMF), a multispecialty medical group serving the San Francisco Bay area. Dr. Yu is Director of Cancer Research at PAMF and graduated from the combined undergraduate and medical school program in medicine at Brown University. His residency was at St. Luke's-Roosevelt Medical Center in New York City, where he was Chief Resident. After a fellowship at Mount Sinai Medical Center, Dr. Yu completed a post-doctoral fellowship at Memorial Sloan-Kettering Cancer Center in the laboratory of Dr. John Mendelsohn. He is board certified in both medical oncology and hematology. He has served as President of the Association of Northern California Oncologists, Chief of Medicine at El Camino Hospital in Mountain View, member of the Board of Directors of Pathways Homecare and Hospice, and is a member of the Audit Committee of the Cancer and Leukemia Group B (CALGB). He is currently a member of the board of directors of the American Society of Clinical Oncology (ASCO) and Chair of the ASCO HIT Work Group. Past ASCO activities have included Chair of the Clinical Practice Committee; member of the Cancer Research, Information Technology, Grant Selection, Audit and Nominating Committees; Chair of the Best of ASCO San Francisco 2005; Chair ASCO EHR Symposium 2009; Annual Meeting Educational Session Chair 2007, 2009, and 2010; and faculty of the Clinical Trials for the Community Oncology Team Workshop 2005. Dr. Yu has served as co-chair of the Commission for Certification of Health Information Technology (CCHIT) Oncology work group, co-chair of the AMA-RAND Clinical Decision Support Oncology work group under contract to the Office of the National Coordinator for Health Information Technology, and co-chair of the ASCO-NCI CORE project, and has participated in several IOM health information technology workshops.

Appendix C

Registered Workshop Attendees

Patrick Archdeacon
Medical Officer
Center for Drug Evaluation and
    Research
U.S. Food and Drug
    Administration

Deborah Ascheim
Associate Professor, Clinical
    Director of Research, InCHOIR
Mount Sinai School of Medicine

Christopher Beardmore
Chief Executive Officer
Translational Research
    Management, LLC

Stefano Bertuzzi
Director, Office of Science Policy,
    Planning and Communications
National Institutes of Mental
    Health

Sue Bogner
Chief Scientist
Institute for the Study of Human
    Error, LLC

Pamela Bradley
Director, Science Policy
American Association for Cancer
    Research

Linda Brady
Director, Division of Neuroscience
    and Basic Behavioral Science
National Institute of Mental
    Health

P. J. Brooks
Health Science Administrator
Office of Rare Diseases Research
National Institutes of Health

Steven Brotman
Senior Vice President, Payment
and Health Care Delivery
Policy
AdvaMed

Suanna Bruinooge
Director, Research Policy
American Society of Clinical
Oncology

Barbara Buch
U.S. Food and Drug
Administration

Liza Bundesen
Acting Chief, Science Policy and
Evaluation Branch
Office of Science Policy, Planning,
and Communications
National Institute of Mental
Health

Robert Califf
Director, Duke Translational
Medicine Institute
Vice Chancellor for Clinical and
Translational Research
Professor of Medicine
Duke University Medical Center

Scott Campbell
Executive Director & CEO
Foundation for the National
Institutes of Health

Tanisha Carino
Senior Vice President
Avalere Health

Kelli Carrington
Lead, Public Affairs
National Institutes of Health
Clinical Center

Christine Carter
Vice President, Scientific Affairs
Society for Women's Health
Research

Dorothy Castille
National Institute on Minority
Health and Health Disparities
National Institutes of Health

Carroll Child
Clinical Research Risk Manager
University of California, San
Francisco

Charles Clayton
Director of Training
American Society of Hematology

Elaine Collier
Senior Advisor to Director
National Center for Research
Resources
National Institutes of Health

Doug Cropper
President and Chief Executive
Officer
Genesis Health System

Dennis Cryer
Chief Medical Officer
CryerHealth

Donna Cryer
CEO
CryerHealth

Ulyana Desiderio
Senior Manager for Scientific
Affairs
American Society of Hematology

Dinora Dominguez
Chief, Patient Recruitment and
    Public Liasion
National Institutes of Health
    Clinical Center

James Doroshow
Director, Division of Cancer
    Treatment and Diagnosis
National Cancer Institute
National Institutes of Health

Jeffrey Drazen
Editor-in-Chief
New England Journal of Medicine

Peggy Eastman
Oncology Times

Paul Eisenberg
Senior Vice President, Global
    Regulatory Affairs and Safety
Amgen Inc.

Lynn Etheredge
Consultant, Rapid Learning
    Project
George Washington University

Gary Filerman
President
Atlas Health Foundation

Louis Fiore
Principal Investigator, VA
    Cooperative Studies Program
Director, VA Cooperative Studies
    Program Coordinating Center,
    Boston
Department of Veterans Affairs

J. Michael Fitzmaurice
Senior Science Advisor for
    Information Technology
Agency for Healthcare Research
    and Quality

Mark Fleury
Associate Director, Science Policy
American Association for Cancer
    Research

Sherine Gabriel
William J. and Charles H. Mayo
    Professor of Medicine &
    Epidemiology, Mayo Medical
    School
Co-Principal Investigator
    and Director of Education,
    Mayo Clinical Center for
    Translational Scientific
    Activities (CTSA)

Jenny Gaffney
Senior Manager
Avalere Health

Elaine Gallin
Principal
QE Philanthropic Advisors

John Gallin
Director, Clinical Center
National Institutes of Health

Annetine Gelijns
Professor of Health Policy
Co-Chair, Department of Health
    Evidence and Policy
Mount Sinai School of Medicine

Robert Giffin
Vice President, Healthcare Policy
    and Reimbursement
Covidien

Andrea Giuffrida
Health Scientist—AAAS Science
    & Technology Policy Fellow
Office of Science Policy
National Institutes of Health

Rashmi Gopal-Srivastava
Director, Extramural Research
    Program
Office of Rare Diseases Research
National Institutes of Health

Jennifer Graff
Research Director, Methods,
    Evidence & Coverage
National Pharmaceutical Council

Cheryl Grandinetti
Health Scientist Policy Analyst
Center for Drug Evaluation and
    Research
U.S. Food and Drug Administration

Candice Griffin
Senior Program Manager
American Society of Clinical
    Oncology

Claudia Grossmann
Program Officer
Institute of Medicine

Kristi Guillory
Senior Policy Analyst
American Cancer Society

Felix Gyi
CEO
Chesapeake IRB

Anthony Hayward
Director, Division for Clinical
    Research Resources
National Center for Research
    Resources
National Institutes of Health

Elina Hemminki
Professor
National Institute for Health and
    Welfare, Helsinki, Finland

Janie Hofacker
Director of Programs
Association of American Cancer
    Institutes

Jeffrey Humphrey
Executive Director
Bristol-Myers Squibb

Ekopimo Ibia
Director
Merck & Co., Inc.

John Iglehart
National Correspondent
New England Journal of Medicine

Rebecca Jackson
Professor and Associate Dean for
    Clinical Research
Director and Principal
    Investigator, OSU Center for
    Clinical and Translational
    Science
The Ohio State University

Michael King Jolly
Senior Vice President
Quintiles Innovation

Rasika Kalamegham
Senior Associate
Pew Charitable Trusts

Petra Kaufmann
Director, Office of Clinical
   Research
National Institute of Neurological
   Disorders and Stroke
National Institutes of Health

Dominick Kennerson
Director
CryerHealth

Steven King
Assistant Executive Director
American College of Radiology

Timothy King
Director
PRA International

Roger Klein
Medical Director, Molecular
   Oncology
Blood Center of Wisconsin,
   Medical College of Wisconsin

Charles Knirsch
Vice President, Clinical Research
Pfizer Inc.

Hon-Sum Ko
Medical Officer
Center for Drug Evaluation and
   Research
U.S. Food and Drug Administration

Kathy Kopnisky
Senior Policy Analyst, Advisor for
   Regulatory Science
Office of Science Policy
National Institutes of Health

Ronald Krall
Associate Fellow
Center for Bioethics
University of Pennsylvania

Judith Kramer
Associate Professor of Medicine,
   Duke University Medical
   Center
Executive Director, Clinical Trials
   Transformation Initiative
   (CTTI)

Steven Krosnick
Program Director
National Cancer Institute
National Institutes of Health

Kelly Lai
Director of Science and
   Regulatory Affairs
Biotechnology Industry
   Organization

Michael Lauer
Director, Division of
   Cardiovascular Sciences
National Heart, Lung, and Blood
   Institute
National Institutes of Health

David Leventhal
Director, Clinical Innovation
Pfizer Inc.

Shao-Lee Lin
Executive Medical Director
Amgen Inc.

Bryan Luce
Senior Vice President, Science
Policy
United BioSource Corporation

Kelsey Mace
Program Coordinator
American Society of Clinical
Oncology

Diane Maloney
Associate Director for Policy
Center for Biologics Evaluation
and Research
U.S. Food and Drug Administration

Michael Marcarelli
Director, Division of Bioresearch
Monotoring
Office of Compliance, Center
for Devices and Radiological
Health
U.S. Food and Drug Administration

Karen Margolis
Professor of Medicine, University
of Minnesota Medical School
Director of Clinical Research
HealthPartners Research
Foundation

Paula McKeever
Senior Policy Coordinator
Center for Drug Evaluation and
Research
U.S. Food and Drug Administration

Marissa Miller
Chief, Advanced Technologies
and Surgery Branch
National Heart, Lung, and Blood
Institute
National Institutes of Health

Carol Mimura
Assistant Vice Chancellor for
Intellectual Property &
Industry Research Alliances
(IPIRA)
University of California, Berkeley

Briggs Morrison
Senior Vice President
Worldwide Medical Excellence
Pfizer Inc.

Catherine Muha
Public Health Advisor
National Cancer Institute
National Institutes of Health

Sharon Murphy
Scholar-in-Residence
National Cancer Policy Forum
Institute of Medicine

Richard Murray
Vice President, Global Center for
Scientific Affairs
Office of the Chief Medical
Officer
Merck & Co., Inc.

Elizabeth Ness
Nurse Consultant
National Cancer Institute
National Institutes of Health

Martha Nolan
Vice President, Public Policy
Society for Women's Health
    Research

Ann O'Mara
Program Director
National Cancer Institute
National Institutes of Health

Keiko Ono
Senior Program Associate
National Research Council

John Orloff
Chief Medical Officer and
    Senior Vice President, Global
    Development, US Medical &
    Drug Regulatory Affairs
Novartis Pharmaceuticals
    Corporation

Maggie Owner
Government Affiars Consultant
Lewis-Burke Associates LLC

Rose Mary Padberg
Public Health Advisor
National Cancer Institute
National Institutes of Health

Linda Parreco
Public Health Advisor
National Cancer Institute
National Institutes of Health

Gary Persinger
Consultant
National Pharmaceutical Council

Richard Platt
Professor, Harvard Medical
    School
Co-Chair, Clinical Effectiveness
    Research Innovation
    Collaboration
IOM Roundtable on Value and
    Science-Driven Health Care

Laura Povlich
AAAS Congressional Fellow
Representative Sandy Levin

Mary Purucker
National Center for Research
    Resources
National Institutes of Health

Elizabeth Rach
Scientist
Cato Research Ltd.

Ihor Rak
Vice President, Clinical
    Neuroscience
AstraZeneca

Domenic Reda
Director
VA Cooperative Studies Program
    Coordinating Center

Stephanie Reffey
Research Science Manager
Susan G. Komen for the Cure

Theodore Reiss
Research Professor of Medicine
Vanderbilt

John Reppas
Director of Public Policy
Neurotechnology Industry
    Organization

Gloria Romanelli
Senior Director
American College of Radiology

Patrick Rooney
Co-Founder
Bionymity, Inc.

Jean Rouleau
Scientific Director, Institute of
    Circulatory and Respiratory
    Health
Canadian Institutes of Health
    Research

Arthur Rubenstein
Professor, Department of
    Medicine, Division of
    Endocrinology
Raymond and Ruth Perelman
    School of Medicine
University of Pennsylvania

Emily Rubinstein
Manager, Data Analytics
Context Matters

Richard Rudick
Hazel Prior Hostetler Chair of
    Neurology, Cleveland Clinic
Professor of Medicine, Cleveland
    Clinic Lerner College of
    Medicine
Case Western Reserve University

Deborah Runkle
Senior Program Associate
American Association for the
    Advancement of Science

Jody Sachs
Program Officer
National Center for Research
    Resources
National Institutes of Health

Chas Scammell
Director, New York
    Pharmaceutical Practice
Milliman

Amber Hartman Scholz
Assistant Executive Director
President's Council of Advisors
    on Science and Technology
    & Office of Science and
    Technology Policy

Jeff Schomisch
Senior Managing Editor
Guide to Good Clinical Practice

Kevin Schulman
Professor of Medicine and
    Gregory Mario and Jeremy
    Mario Professor of Business
    Administration
Duke University School of
    Medicine and the Fuqua School
    of Business

Talisha Searcy
Program Analyst
Office of Inspector General, Office
    of Evaluation and Inspections
U.S. Department of Health and
    Human Services

Joe Selby
Executive Director
Patient-Centered Outcomes
    Research Institute

Lisa Shapiro
Associate Director, Clinical
    Program Management
Astellas Pharma Global
    Development

Rachel Sherman
Associate Director for Medical
    Policy
Center for Drug Evaluation and
    Research
U.S. Food and Drug Administration

Mark Smith
Policy Counsel
National Coalition for Cancer
    Research

Phillip Smith
Director, Planning, Evaluation
    and Research
Indian Health Service

Heather Snyder
Senior Associate Director,
    Scientific Grants
Alzheimer's Association

Anil Srivastava
Director
Open Health Systems Laboratory

Scott Steele
Director, Research Alliances
University of Rochester

Kathleen Stratton
Project Director
Pew Charitable Trusts

Tibor Szentendrei
Senior Clinical Research Scientist
KAI Research, Inc.

Carmen Tamayo
R&D Consultant
HeteroGeneity, LLC

Jacob Tenai
Director
Orphan Child Africa
    Organization

Umesh Thakkar
Senior General Engineer
U.S. Government Accountability
    Office

Douglas Throckmorton
Deputy Director, Center for Drug
    Evaluation & Research
U.S. Food and Drug Administration

Janet Tobias
President Sierra/Tango
    Productions
Ikana Media

Sean Tunis
President & CEO
Center for Medical Technology
    Policy

Kathleen Uhl
Deputy Director, Office of
    Medical Policy
Center for Drug Evaluation and
    Research
U.S. Food and Drug Administration

Jill Wechsler
Washington Editor
Pharmaceutical Executive magazine

Neil Weisfeld
New Associates, LLC

Neil Weissman
President
MedStar Health Research
    Institute

Clarissa Wittenberg
Consultant
European Organization for
    Research and Treatment of
    Cancer

Hui-Hsing Wong
Medical Officer
Assistant Secretary for Planning
    and Evaluation
U.S. Department of Health and
    Human Services

Alastair Wood
Partner & Managing Director
Symphony Capital LLC

Janet Woodcock
Director
Center for Drug Evaluation and
    Research
U.S. Food and Drug Administration

Clyde Yancy
Magerstadt Professor of
    Medicine, Chief, Division of
    Cardiology
Feinberg School of Medicine,
    Northwestern University

Tara Yazinski
Advocate
National Fibromyalgia and
    Chronic Pain Association

John Yeh
Professor
Massachusetts General Hospital,
    Harvard

Peter Yu
Oncologist, Palo Alto Medical
    Foundation
Chair, Electronic Health Record
    Working Group
American Society of Clinical
    Oncology

Deborah Zarin
Director, ClinicalTrials.gov
National Library of Medicine

Paul Zimmet
Research Advocate
Parkinson's Disease Foundation

Bram Zuckerman
Director
Division of Cardiovascular
    Devices
U.S. Food and Drug Administration

Appendix D

Discussion Paper[1]

The Clinical Trials Enterprise in the United States: A Call for Disruptive Innovation

Robert M. Califf, Duke University Medical Center; Gary L. Filerman, Atlas Health Foundation; Richard K. Murray, Merck & Co., Inc.; and Michael Rosenblatt, Merck & Co., Inc.[2]

INTRODUCTION

Over the past decade, the symbiotic relationship between the clinical trials enterprise (CTE) and the health care delivery system has been subject to increasing amounts of stress. During this period, the CTE has primarily focused on process improvement, seeking to create and maintain procedures and data systems that can satisfy a regulatory environment concerned with specific research procedures. These efforts have driven up the cost of research and left the CTE increasingly out of sync with the health care delivery system.

At the same time, there have been many significant changes in the health care delivery system, changes largely concerned with organization, quality improvement, operational efficiency, and error reduction

---

[1] The views expressed in this discussion paper are those of the authors and not necessarily of the authors' organizations or of the Institute of Medicine. The paper is intended to help inform and stimulate discussion. It has not been subjected to the review procedures of the Institute of Medicine and is not a report of the Institute of Medicine or of the National Research Council.

[2] Participants in the activities of the IOM Forum on Drug Discovery, Development, and Translation. This discussion paper was presented in draft form at the Forum's November 2011 workshop, Envisioning a Transformed Clinical Trials Enterprise in the United States: Establishing an Agenda for 2020, and finalized by the authors following the workshop. The authors would like to thank David Davis, Jeffrey Drazen, Ronald Krall, Samuel Nussbaum, Neil Weissman, and Marcus Wilson for their comments and suggestions on draft versions of this paper.

and patient safety. Despite significant rhetoric (particularly in the United States) about "learning health systems" (Institute of Medicine [IOM], 2007), the CTE and the health care delivery system have continued to diverge. This situation is undesirable both because research done within such a partitioned, parallel system may not be broadly generalizable and because the cost of maintaining parallel systems limits our ability to address critical gaps in knowledge.

The end result of the widening separation between research and health care delivery will be a serious deficit in new knowledge about the benefits and risks of specific drugs and devices in medical practice at a time when biological knowledge is expanding exponentially (see Figure 1) and warnings about the unsustainability of the system continue to escalate (IOM, 2008). This systemic divergence, in turn, deprives providers of reliable evidence upon which to base their practices, deprives patients of the expected return on research investments in science and medicine, and deprives policy makers of a rational basis for choosing one course of action over another.

The scope and pace of change in the overall health system will only increase as we enter the next decade, exacerbating the undesirable separation of research and practice. There is thus an urgent need to develop policies that will mitigate current stresses and increase CTE efficiency and effectiveness by expeditiously forming a deliberate plan to align the CTE and the emerging health care delivery system. Such an effort will require a new assertion of the societal values that underlie the CTE, a clarification of the objectives of such a plan, and accommodations on the parts of both the CTE and the health care delivery system to accomplish those objectives.

A decade ago, the National Institutes of Health (NIH) embarked upon a major effort to reshape the future of biomedical research. This framework for change, called the NIH Roadmap (Zerhouni, 2003), articulated a vision for clinical research in which each of more than 300 million Americans would have his or her own electronic health record (EHR). If individuals so chose (assuming appropriate privacy and confidentiality protections), the information in these EHRs could be used for research, and patients and their families would be joined together in networks that could answer critical questions about prevention and treatment. The fabric of constantly-accruing data would form the basis of a learning health system in which randomized trials could be performed by inserting randomization into the routine delivery of health care. This revolutionary approach would allow the rapid and definitive development of evidence at a relatively low cost.

Although this vision from a decade ago has not been achieved, much of it is within reach by 2020. Consolidations of service delivery and insurance organizations are changing the context of practice. Technological limitations are being overcome, disease-oriented networks and voluntary health organizations are evolving, and modern medical informatics is enabling the aggregation, classification, indexing, and analysis of information in volumes that were unimaginable a decade ago. Unfortunately, at the same time these tools are emerging, the CTE is increasingly being cordoned off from the rapidly-evolving, information-intensive world of medical practice. This paper provides a roadmap for integrating the clinical trials and health care delivery systems in ways that will improve the efficiency and effectiveness of both.

Current Status of the Clinical Trials Enterprise

The passage of the Food and Drug Administration (FDA) Amendment Act in 2007 (FDA, 2007) mandated the registration of most clinical trials involving medical products approved for use in the United States. The resulting increase in the number of trials registered and the quality of the information provided to entities such as ClinicalTrials.gov has afforded us a new opportunity to assess the state of the overall CTE.

When we examine these data, several significant patterns are manifest. First, the vast majority of clinical research comprises tiny trials performed on small numbers of patients (62 percent of studies plan to accrue fewer than 100 participants; 96 percent have a projected accrual of <1,000) (Califf et al. [in review]). Second, the majority of trials are sponsored by academic health centers (AHCs) and are focused on disease mechanisms, or are phase 1 and 2 studies sponsored by industry. The majority of research participants, however, are enrolled in industry-sponsored phase 2, 3, or 4 trials that are fewer but larger in size and increasingly globalized (Glickman et al., 2009). Third, relatively few trials are asking questions that directly address critical decision points in clinical practice.

A typical clinical trial today depends on the recruitment of investigators who, in turn, recruit trial participants and oversee the conduct of the research protocol. There is, however, no assurance that the recruited participants are sufficiently representative of broader populations to allow generalization of trial results. Further, these trials are often conducted at professional clinical trial sites that produce clean data, but at the cost of divorcing the trial from clinical care. At the same time, we now have multiple integrated health systems, including not only well-known health management organizations (HMOs) and the Department of Veterans Affairs (VA) system, but also numerous integrated health systems (IHSs) that possess data warehouses capable of supporting the selection of research participants in a much more systematic fashion.

These problems are compounded by a decline in the number of U.S. investigators, while at the same time the total number of clinical trials worldwide has nearly doubled in the last decade (Getz, 2005). This decline also coincides with a rapid expansion of the offshoring of clinical research activities, a particularly worrisome trend (Califf, 2011; Kim et al., 2011). In this context, "offshoring" of trials refers to the movement of research away from the United States purely because of the excess cost and difficulty of conducting research domestically, including long start-up times, slow recruitment, and high rates of non-adherence and withdrawal of consent. Offshoring is not a synonym for globalization, which allows many countries and cultures to participate in research and which we regard as a positive development for all diseases. Globalization of clinical research can be particularly beneficial when the research addresses neglected diseases (Bollyky, 2011) or major chronic diseases that may have a different outcome or treatment effect with different genetic backgrounds or patterns of clinical care than those found in the United States.

Offshoring is a concern because it diminishes synergies between basic and clinical research that are vital to translational research, and because it weakens the interface with industry that speeds advances in drugs and devices made available to the American public. Furthermore, research performed in different populations or under different conditions may not be fully generalizable unless particular care is taken. And while the NIH Roadmap vision calls for a seamless and efficient integration of research and practice, in reality we see that the focus on efficiency in practice has led to the view that research is a source of additional expense and burdensome administrative and regulatory commitments (Califf, 2009). At the same time, when clinical research is not integrated with practice, its focus on efficiency in isolation from other factors distances it further from the environment crucial to producing generalizable results.

PART I: ORGANIZATION OF HEALTH SERVICES IN 2020

This section describes our vision of the health systems of 2020. In health services, demography is destiny. At the largest scale, demographic patterns drive a substantial portion of the demand for services. Less obvious, however, is the manner in which American demography mandates the organization of the services that respond to that demand, how and by whom services are paid for, and who provides the services. The U.S. Census Bureau estimates that by 2020 there will be more than 341 million Americans, of whom nearly 55 million (16 percent) will be 65 years of age or older. Among these will be an estimated 135,000 centenarians (U.S. Census Bureau, 2008). The population of the country as a whole will be ethnically diverse; this will be especially true for those under the age of 20. Most patient and provider interactions will take place in the context of managing chronic conditions—chiefly depression, cancers, cardiovascular disease, diabetes, arthritis, asthma, and Alzheimer's disease.

Throughout their lifetimes, most Americans will either be enrolled in or anticipating enrollment in an IHS that will provide all or nearly all of their health care. By 2020, there will be substantial but uneven progress toward establishing the IHS as the dominant form of health care organization, particularly in urban settings. Elements of IHS implementation will be in place in most communities.

The typical IHS is community hospital–centered and oriented toward providing primary care. Integration is driven by enrollment, bundled payment, EHRs, and standardized health care. It serves an enrolled (i.e., defined) population. It is further defined by the scope of and coordination among the comprehensive services that comprise its network, including directly owned or contracted multi-specialty medical group practices, ambulatory care centers (including imaging, walk-in "retail" clinics, employee wellness facilities, rehabilitation centers, etc.), home health agencies, nursing homes, extended care facilities, and hospital- and home-based hospice services within its primary service area. Most IHSs are affiliated with local public health departments and community health centers. All IHSs have collaborative agreements with AHCs for education and research support. The IHS and/or affiliated group practices serves as the locus of medical homes and accountable care organizations.

Integrated health care organizations and their affiliated service organizations either employ or contract with a substantial majority of health care providers, including physicians, nurses, advanced-practice nurses, physician assistants, clinical social workers, and psychologists. Pharmacists are engaged in provider and patient counseling across the system. Although IHSs provide comprehensive data, patients/customers and their families switch from one IHS to another, with the result that interoperability is an indispensible characteristic of any viable data system.

Health care professionals have a strong sense of identity with the IHS, which is the focus of much of their professional activity. There is also a high degree of alignment between system objectives and professional expectations and roles that is achieved through recruitment, position and role description, promotion, remuneration, and incentives. The objective of implementing a culture of patient-centered care through the optimal deployment of appropriate competencies is reflected in the organization of teams that respond to the patient's changing needs.

The EHR can be characterized as the clinical and administrative core of the IHS. It is designed to meet both administrative and clinical needs and employs nationally standardized interoperability and nomenclature. The scope of "meaningful use" of EHR technology has been expanded to embrace and incentivize research. Empowered by virtualization, the

EHR is designed to enable preventive, clinical, and supportive services throughout an enrollee's life. The development and maturation of EHR technologies promise to make practicable the application of genetic information to medical practice. The EHR is also designed to provide the continuous aggregate data that are essential for assessing the health of the enrolled population, continually improving the quality of care throughout the IHS, and supporting clinical research and professional education. Of paramount importance, however, is the fact that the EHR enables the system, the provider, and the researcher to follow up with the patient over time. Large population-based real-time evidence is the product of aggregated health system databases. Randomization is facilitated through super computer–based virtually-integrated information systems that merge administrative and clinical data from multiple sources. The virtually-integrated networks, spanning providers and payers, make it possible to enroll individuals in trials and to follow them going forward. The magnitude of the databases and the power of the tools make possible analyses that are responsive to the cultural diversity of the study populations.

The EHR is first initiated when the patient enrolls or enters any of the component organizations and services. Integrated with web-based mobile technology, the EHR "follows" the patient home, issuing reminders and monitoring compliance, as well as capturing incidents and wellness indicators (FasterCures, 2005). In 2020, there is wide public recognition that research is an integral component of community-based practice. The basic compact between the patient and the provider community is that every patient is a potential contributor to research. It is assumed that the patient record may be used for research in a de-identified data system. The patient-oriented part of the EHR is owned by the patient and is accessible only by the patient or by family members and providers to whom the patient grants access. Special permission is required to use such information in research projects that could potentially identify the individual.

The maintenance and improvement of professional competence is an objective of all IHSs and defines them, in the terms of an earlier IOM report, as "learning health systems" (IOM, 2011a). The formal relationships with providers across all participating settings as well as the aggregate clinical and administrative data generated by the EHR provide the foundation for feedback and for rigorous and sustained continuing education. Every health care delivery site is a learning site, providing continuing health education (CHE) that includes point-of-care reminders, links to clinical practice guidelines, and other online resources. This is in addition to traditional CME activities that are at once targeted to the objectives of the IHS and to the need for education where it is most effective—the point of patient engagement.

In 2020 the professional specialty societies, providing leadership for knowledge, are one of the most influential factors moving research participation into the definition of successful practice. Research participation is highlighted and promoted in the educational programs, publications, and recogitions of the societies. The societies support research directly by maintaining registries of clinical experience to which they have unique access and through fellowships that enable community-based practitioners to gain research experience. Board-certification requirements recognize research and particularly translation skills.

Academic health centers are integrally related to IHSs. The missions and priorities of AHCs have been clarified to distinguish between those with a substantial investment in basic and translational research, and those that are primarily focused on education and service. The more comprehensive of the former have been designated as academic health science systems (AHSSs) (Dzau, et al. 2010). All AHSSs are organized to serve as research sites for enrollment in observational studies and interventional trials. All IHSs are affiliated with an AHC, which could be an AHSS, which serves them as a resource for education and clinical research through an affiliated IHS office or department. In most cases, the affiliated academic centers have access to the IHS databases for the purpose of maintaining registries and conducting collaborative projects.

A fundamental element undergirding mature electronic health and medical records is the application of an ontology that permits the same terms to be used for describing clinical phenomena and for billing; they also form the basis for quality measurement and for providing adjustments for severity of illness when efficiency measures are assessed. These same terms will also constitute the fundamental "vocabulary" for both observational research databases and randomized controlled trials (RCTs). When needed, additional data elements are added for more detailed investigation and randomization is applied to the record. While the nation has yet to reach this envisioned state of health system integration and effective use of the EHR, the implementation of national health care reform legislation and the efforts of organizations to display their accountability for health care outcomes and costs will likely bring us closer to this stated vision.

PART II: THE FUTURE OF CLINICAL RESEARCH

Controlled clinical trials are the essential cornerstone of modern evidence-based medical care and health practice. Although multiple types of information are needed to fully inform practice, the interventional clinical trial (ICT) plays a particularly critical role. When we view scientific studies as a continuum, we see that they are translated into treatments through a series of steps, beginning with preclinical research that evolves into early-phase clinical trials designed to assess safety and demonstrate proof-of-concept for on-target and off-target effects. Successful interventions (drugs, devices, behavioral strategies) are next evaluated using controlled trials to determine whether the balance of risks and benefits merits the marketing of the technology or intervention. When such studies are robust, practice guidelines can be developed to guide clinical decision making; when they are definitive, guidelines can be distilled into performance measures to assess the quality of practice. At the heart of this paradigm is the measurement of process and outcomes, combined with the use of the measurement system to guide continuous education of practitioners and to assess therapeutic deficits that require new interventions to overcome.

When the effects of an intervention are modest (as is typically the case), randomization provides the most reliable method for determining the true effect of the intervention compared with an alternative. The first known description of an interventional trial is Lind's 18th-century account of using fruit to combat scurvy (Lind, 1753). Following Fisher's pioneering demonstration of randomization in a series of agricultural experiments in the 1920s (Fisher, 1926), the first randomized clinical trial was conducted by the British Medical Research Council to evaluate streptomycin for tuberculosis in 1946 (Medical Research Council, 1948). In the 1960s the NIH became the dominant force in developing clinical trials methodologies (Coronary Drug Project Research Group, 1973) and in 1962, following passage of the Kefauver-Harris Drug Amendments, the FDA took the position that efficacy must be established prior to the marketing of drugs (FDA, 2006). As a result of these developments, the RCT was adopted as the standard by which efficacy was determined. Soon, regulatory agencies in other countries joined in, and the majority of research participants were enrolled in trials sponsored by industry and intended to develop or evaluate drugs or devices. In the 1990s the CTE globalized, spurred by the simultaneous expansion of medical technology development together with the global need to understand the effects of health interventions (as well as any associated economic and scientific benefits) in all societies.

A major problem in the field of clinical research is the current absence of a standard ontology that adequately encompasses its activities, rendering it difficult to characterize the state of the enterprise. Common metrics must be based on common definitions so that valid comparisons can be made and policy decisions are based on solid evidence. This problem is illustrated by the multiple definitions of the term "clinical trial." For the purposes of this report, we have adopted the definition used by the ClinicalTrials.gov registry: "biomedical or health-related research studies in human beings that follow a pre-defined protocol. Interventional studies are those in which the research subjects are assigned by the investigator to a treatment or other intervention, and their outcomes are measured" (National Institutes of Health, 2007). This broad definition thus includes nonrandomized interventions but excludes registries that simply measure practice, as well as research confined to databases. As the clinical research ontology develops, better classification will be key to accurately measuring the progress of the enterprise by comparing the same types of studies and methods over time.

Currently, more than 330 clinical trials are registered every week with the ClinicalTrials.gov registry, which now contains data on more than 110,000 studies. In reviewing data from ClinicalTrials.gov, the CTE is revealed as highly complex, with research studies fulfilling a wide variety of purposes (see Table 1). As we noted earlier, the majority of clinical trials are small, conducted in AHSSs, and sponsored either by the federal government (typically through the NIH) or funded internally by the academic organization. However, the vast majority of *patients* are enrolled in industry-sponsored trials, due to academic trials' small size and the fact that they are typically not intended to inform practice; rather, academic trials are oriented toward elucidating biological mechanisms or developing pilot data. However, industry resembles academic research in one respect: it conducts many more small, early-phase trials than it does large studies intended to inform practice. While trials are conducted in all disease areas, the distribution is dominated by cancer, cardiovascular medicine, and mental health. Both across disease areas and within specialty areas, it is clear that trial portfolios do not match public health or community medical practice needs in terms of either magnitude or urgency.

Historically, the United States has been a dominant presence in clinical research, but there is growing concern that the enterprise is in decline. There is ample evidence that U.S. trials are becoming more expensive (DeVol et al., 2011). Worse, 90 percent fail to meet enrollment goals, and additional evidence points to disillusionment among American investigators (Getz, 2005). The rate of attrition among U.S. investigators is increasing, even among experienced researchers with strong track records of productivity, while 45 percent of first-time investigators abandon the field after their first trial. The system has become so inefficient that even the NIH is offshoring clinical trials at a substantial rate (Califf, 2011; Kim et al., 2011), using taxpayer funding to conduct trials in countries with less expensive and more efficient CTEs, despite concerns about generalizability as noted above.

While the CTE is in decline in the United States, the need for trials, paradoxically, is increasingly well-recognized. Recent reports indicate that fewer than 15 percent of major recommendations in clinical practice guidelines in infectious disease (Lee and Vielemeyer, 2011) and cardio-vascular disease (Tricoci et al., 2009) are based on solid evidence. Recent failures to perform proper trials have led to public health hazards after drugs were developed and marketed without proper supporting evi-dence. The wide-scale use of antiarrhythmic drugs provides a sentinel example: the CAST Trial (Pratt and Moye, 1990) demonstrated that a treatment that was being used to prevent death was actually causing excess mortality. Similarly, hormone replacement therapy (HRT) was thought to reduce cardiovascular disease until the HERS Trial (Hulley et al., 1998) and the Women's Health Initiative (Rossouw et al., 2002) demonstrated an excess hazard for cardiovascular events with HRT. Most recently, high-dose erythropoietin appeared to provide substantial ben-efit in anemia related to renal failure and cancer, and clinical practice guidelines touted its use. But when controlled trials were finally done, high-dose erythropoiesis-stimulating agents were found to cause excess cardiovascular events (Bennet et al., 2008; FDA, 2011; Pfeffer et al., 2009; Singh et al., 2006). Never has the need for properly controlled interven-tional trials been so clear.

The decline of the U.S. CTE has been noticed by other countries, which are moving rapidly to fill in the gap. The United Kingdom has recently published a national strategy aimed at gaining a larger market share of clinical trials (The Academy of Medical Sciences, 2011) and has made research a primary mission of the National Health Service. Canada has developed a national plan (Canadian Institutes of Health Research, 2011) and China and India are focused on increasing their participation in clinical trials (Gupta and Padhy, 2011; Jia, 2005). At the same time, many countries are providing incentives for industry to locate clinical trials in their countries.

As we note above, we regard globalization of clinical trials as an important positive trend, but the motivating factor should be to provide population- and culture-specific medical evidence to inform local practice. If globalization takes place merely because the United States cannot enroll research participants or has priced itself out of the market, the net result may prove negative. Having countries assume a low-cost vendor status in circumstances where their own populations may not benefit from the research is also troubling from an ethical perspective.

Substantial evidence indicates that the fundamental problem is not rooted in the attitudes of the U.S. public. Although there appears to be variation among socioeconomic and ethnic groups, the public in general places high value on both research in general and clinical research in par-ticular. The majority of Americans report that they would either certainly or most likely participate in research if asked (Getz, 2011). Additionally, an overwhelming majority of those who participate in clinical trials find them to be a positive experience and report that they would do it again. Rather, the problem is not with people but with the health care system—patients are not being asked to participate and many barriers exist (IOM, 2011b).

Because of these challenges, we believe that the CTE can and must be improved and integrated with the evolving health care delivery system as part of an essential evolution toward the learning health system envisioned by the IOM (2007). The CTE can be envisioned as four overlapping enterprises, which we refer to as "laboratories" to emphasize the vast needs that remain to be addressed by the continuing evolution of the entire system. These laboratories share a common fabric of methods, but are different enough that specialized training and education will be needed, intensive methodological work will be required, and investments must be made to produce results that can revolutionize our understanding of how to better prevent, manage, and treat disease.

The Innovator's Lab

The majority of clinical trials will continue to enroll small numbers of research participants to address biological hypotheses, to develop initial evidence about the mechanisms of action of drugs, devices, and other interventions, or to develop preliminary evidence of their risk–benefit profile. We believe that the world of phase 1 units and academic studies must be combined into a much more effective approach to human systems biology. This new system should be highly networked, enabling researchers to leverage major advances in genetics, genomics, and biomarkers.

Because studies of biological mechanisms and early studies of new therapies require intensive measurements in human volunteers, these studies should be performed in an environment separate from the health care delivery system. Recent evaluation has implicated both a failure to fully engage the biological target of therapy as well as "off-target" effects in the high rate of attrition characteristic of early-phase trials. Also, when late-phase failures are evaluated, off-target effects frequently emerge as the cause. Systems biological measurements, in which multiple biological outcomes can be monitored simultaneously, promise better characterization of on-target effects as well as better identification of off-target effects.

The environment for this type of research should be intensive in terms of highly qualified staff and sophisticated data-management capabilities. Because the studied populations will either be 1) normal volunteers or 2) patients with a disease of interest exposed to a new drug or device and/ or undergoing intensive measurement, the most effective environment will likely be found within a hospital with advanced emergency care, imaging, and data capabilities.

Currently, these types of studies are either done in commercial "phase 1 units" or academic medical centers funded by the Clinical and Translational Science Awards (CTSA) program (CTSAs, 2011). However, phase 1 units lack sophisticated technologies for measuring biological mechanisms and are typically not collocated within a hospital. Academic centers are limited as well: they typically have inefficient units that are focused on specific investigator needs and not on throughput and sponsor needs.

The Traditional Lab

Even under the new system, there will still be a need for traditional trials designed to determine the efficacy of an intervention or to assess the balance of risks and benefits in carefully defined populations. Although these studies are labor-intensive and expensive, they are indispensible in determining whether a technology has any significant effect compared with placebo or standard treatment. In some cases, these studies should be done in the context of clinical care (e.g., when research participants are acutely ill). In other circumstances, they can be done in stand-alone research centers designed to effectively administer experimental treatment and collect extensive data on efficacy measures and adverse events.

There is overlap between the traditional lab and the health care delivery lab, especially in comparative-effectiveness research (CER). As the demand for comparative evidence grows, so too will the need for trials with pragmatic features that are carefully controlled, may be blinded, and are performed in the context of clinical practice (Eisenstein et al., 2008; Tunis et al., 2010; Yusuf et al., 2008).

One example of the first type of efficacy study can be seen in the setting of acute myocardial infarction (AMI). Patients presenting in the midst of a life-threatening emergency such as AMI must be enrolled in studies while at the same time receiving urgent medical care. For at least the first 1,500 patients enrolled on a trial of a new treatment, there must be intensive collection of adverse events to ensure that an unexpected toxicity (or benefit) is not occurring.

An example of the second type of efficacy study would be a trial of a new treatment for seasonal allergies, in which there is no reason to burden the health care delivery system with people who can elect to participate in a trial of a less serious condition. While this type of study could be done in primary care practices, it might also be done most efficiently in stand-alone research centers divorced from the pressures of the practice environment. As trials methodology advances, the efficiency afforded by a study site outside clinical practice must be weighed against the generalizability of the findings.

The Health Care Delivery System as Laboratory

The central premise of this paper is that achieving the highest potential of clinical research depends upon the incorporation of clinical research into the broad scope of practice of health care delivery. Doctors, nurses, and other providers should regard it as their business to generate evidence as well as to translate it into practice. This research should include evaluation of the risks and benefits of technologies, the assessment of methods of delivering interventions at the point of care, as well as organizational aspects of health care.

The critical need for knowledge to guide diagnosis, assessment, and treatment of disease cannot be met by the current divided system, with its redundant domains for personnel and data collection. We have a significant window of opportunity arising from the development of EHRs and the drive to collect well-defined data for quality improvement and population health endeavors. If data from integrated health systems can be used for clinical trials as well as quality improvement/population health, the incremental cost of clinical trials could be reduced significantly.

In addition to the development of standardized data collection and ontologies, this transformation requires the adoption of and financial support for knowledge generation as a fundamental value of the health care delivery system. Providers, as well as patients and their families, must be made aware of the cost in lives and disability that inevitably accompanies failure to define benefits and risks in the context of health care. If we successfully cultivate this awareness, obtaining consent and inserting randomization into the treatment paradigm will not be regarded as an impediment to efficiency; instead, they will be viewed as essential elements of ethical and appropriate health care delivery. The immediate results of such a fundamental change to the system will be a dramatic increase in the amount and quality of evidence available to inform practice, combined with a fine-tuning of the system to achieve best practices as a matter of course.

As mentioned above, there is overlap between the traditional lab and the clinical practice lab in the area of CER. These regions of overlap will evolve further as data warehouses are used to conduct postmarketing studies of drug and device safety (Behrman et al., 2011).

The Community Engagement Lab

Many interventions that have a potentially great impact on health either do not involve the health care delivery system or do so only peripherally. Daunting questions about disease prevention, managing a healthful lifestyle, and living with chronic illness require the application of a variety of methods, but clinical trials should be an element of the repertoire.

One important type of study will formally assess approaches to prevention or behavioral intervention in chronic disease. While the health care delivery system may be involved, the majority of a given intervention may well take place in homes, schools, or neighborhoods. This research will require adoption of principles of community engagement, so that the needs of individuals and their communities are understood, allowing them to participate with full knowledge of the methods and rationales for specific clinical trials.

An essential method in this major area of research will be cluster randomization, an approach that randomly allocates "units" to different interventional strategies. These units may include clinics, hospitals, neighborhoods, or communities. Cluster randomization may provide the most efficient method for determining optimal public health policies.

A new and rapidly evolving approach to clinical trials is being developed by voluntary health organizations and other entities that have pioneered using the Internet for this purpose, without significant health delivery system involvement or control. In fact, the use of patient-reported outcomes (PROs), both through voluntary health organizations and through IHS records, provides a basis for incorporating subjective elements into the research paradigm, so that the impact of interventions on quality of life can be assessed in a systematic, generalizable manner.

PART III: SPECIFIC STEPS TO ACHIEVE THE VISION: THE INNOVATOR'S AND TRADITIONAL LABS

Revival of these arenas in the United States will depend upon successful reinvigoration of the NIH's clinical research efforts and the development of effective public–private partnerships to drive research. The newly formed National Center for Advancing Translational Sciences (NCATS) (Collins, 2011) has the potential to catalyze the many elements of the system that must be combined to achieve successful transformation. In particular, the Innovator's Lab would be stimulated by networking of the former general clinical research centers (GCRCs) and the development of a common informatics infrastructure, with core technologies available for assessing systems biology and linking phenotypic information with genomic and physiological data.

The Traditional Lab should be rejuvenated by linking more efficient traditional research-site functions with the evolving health care delivery lab. Given the higher cost of labor in the United States, the only way to remain competitive in this arena is through innovation in data collection and study procedures. Of note, recent findings demonstrating heterogeneity in treatment effects as a function of the country of enrollment (Mahaffey et al., 2011; O'Connor et al., 2011; Simes et al., 2010) have led the FDA to require more U.S. enrollment for studies of products intended for domestic marketing, so success in this arena is a critical element of the overall plan. Simply offshoring this research is not a viable approach to informing the U.S. population of the best choices with regard to treatment and diagnostic strategies.

How the Vision Can Be Achieved Through the Integrated Health System as Health Care Delivery Laboratory

It is both possible and essential that we expand participation in controlled clinical trials in a cost-effective manner, ensuring that such research reflects the general population, their providers, and the range of settings in the health care delivery system of 2020. However, success will require a new approach to the partnership between the CTE and the health care delivery system, one that builds on the centrality of the emerging IHSs and their access to community-based practitioners and hospitals. Expanding the base of clinical research to include many if not most of the non-academic IHSs will result in important contributions to the vitality of service-delivery systems and to the richness of professional practice in all of the participating entities.

In addition to nurturing clinician research, these Health Care Delivery Laboratories will facilitate the translation of research from the bedside to community practice. And they will also stimulate essential feedback from community practice to academic research, with community-based clinicians being encouraged to initiate and participate in knowledge development. In addition, they will enhance the professional development of clinicians across integrated systems and increase community engagement and support. These learning organizations will provide health professions students with the opportunity to observe the professional and practical benefits of participating in clinical research across the full spectrum of practice settings.

A Practical Roadmap to Implementation

Direction and commitment on the part of health system leadership will be essential to forging this new partnership. Both IHS governance and management leadership must understand and communicate the value added by explicitly building research into the mission, objectives, and strategies of the organization; further, they must be charged with shaping a supportive culture. Their message is that participation in clinical and system-improvement research is an essential dimension of the social compact among the health care delivery system, health care providers, the public, and the scientific enterprises that serve them. We recognize that this definition of scope of practice to include research is disruptive. That is the point. We cannot continue a practice and education pattern that is not optimally responsive to, or aligned with, the needs of science and society.

Research in this context is broadly defined to include clinical trials, but also embraces "a much broader range of investigative methods. These methods include epidemiological observations, clinical observations, quasi-experimental evaluations of natural experiments, time series experiments, case studies of apparently successful projects or organizations, rapid-cycle learning and qualitative studies, either alone or as mixed studies in combinations with quantitative studies" (Kottke et al., 2008). It includes health services and operations research to improve the qualitative and economic performance of the system.

A typical health system mission is "to provide quality of care to the community and contribute to medical knowledge." An example of a specific priority objective of many systems might be to build specialty-service lines such as cardiology and oncology with the aim of becoming the leading center in the region. Participating in research, including clinical trials, is a realistic strategy toward accomplishing that objective, and may in fact be a prerequisite of success.

Incorporating research as a core element of a health system's mission, objectives, and strategies will enhance the system's stature and attract political, community, and financial support. It will also expedite the recruitment of practitioners and other employees who aspire to be associated with an organization at the leading edge of health care development.

A supportive infrastructure, aligned with a culture that values research and education, depends upon the commitment of clinical leadership to implement a research business plan. An important objective of the plan is to provide potential research sponsors with a single portal to the system— one that is responsive to their needs and facilitates system-wide access to practitioner investigators.

A well-developed business plan will address specific goals, resources and their allocation, and the timeline for implementation. It will address how the system will communicate with patients to establish the expectation that they may be invited to participate in clinical research. It will address how the organization can identify, reduce, or remove impediments to practitioner participation and overcome the understandable reluctance of busy providers to engage in the research process.

Research business plans may be implemented at the level of the integrated delivery system, affiliated physician groups, and other community-based entities, or all three, if those entities are well-coordinated. There are medical groups, not affiliated with an academic medical center, that are implementing successful research business plans that focus on clinical trials. These community-based sites, or networks, can enter into agreements with research institutes and contract research organizations (CROs) to recruit patients and implement clinical trial protocols. These groups are profitable and have high levels of practitioner participation and patient enrollment and indicate that active clinical practices outside an academic medical center can successfully add clinical trials to their business plans. We can advance the vision of this paper's Practical Road-map by looking to these groups as learning laboratories.

Small systems and medical groups may establish leadership by broadening the Chief Medical Officer role to include responsibility for research development and possibly for education. Others may create a new position of Research Director, while more complex systems may establish a Research Institute or Department. The designated research leader can encourage practitioners to become involved in research by conducting "tentative ideas" seminars, offering methods coaching, and arranging for mentoring.

The research objective will be further enhanced over time by building research promotion and support into the position descriptions of department heads, practice directors, and chairs, so that individuals are recruited into the organization with that expectation. The incentive system in a community hospital–based system can be designed to recognize research participation, including providing supplementary income and the opportunity for protected time.

Customer-friendly administrative support is a major factor in encouraging investigator-initiated clinical research, as well as expanding practitioner participation in government- and industry-supported clinical trials. Such support includes assistance in proposal writing, ethical review, privacy questions, grant administration, IRB relationships, incident reporting, data management and reporting, and preparation of publications.

Some start-up investments are of course necessary. Assuming that the sponsor's business plan includes appropriate reimbursement, it is likely that a robust clinical research program will be self-supporting, if not profitable. Modest strategic investments will attract and stimulate practitioner interest. These may include small seed grants for proposal development, research assistants, and attendance at meetings. A small fund would also support participation in networks and collaboratives.

The IHS will further its research objectives by celebrating the research participation and accomplishments of practitioner researchers. The national goal of expanding Health Care Delivery Labs will be enhanced if the research initiatives of community-based practitioners in integrated delivery systems lead to those practitioners being recognized as "clinical research associates," thereby positively differentiating them from their peers. Participation in clinical trials and other research can be a focus of presentations within the system and provide a basis for communications to the community, enhancing the message that their health system is a learning organization.

PART IV: IMPLEMENTING THE RESEARCH AGENDA

This vision of disruptive innovation, one that is necessary to transform the challenged 2011 CTE into the robust CTE of 2020, generates researchable questions to be addressed with alacrity by the health services community. These questions reside largely in the domain of health services research (HSR), which has been defined as "a multidisciplinary field of inquiry, both basic and applied, that examines the use, costs, quality, accessibility, delivery, organization, financing and outcomes of health care services" (IOM, 1995).

As implementation of the integrated community-based health system model proceeds, the following questions are examples of the research agenda that is called for:

- What are successful cases of securing health system cultural change and system-wide buy-in?
- What are the specific impediments to change in organizational culture?
- How have each of the impediments been managed?
- What are the financing and costing alternatives and their implications?
- How have the systems that have adopted a research agenda organized to implement it?
- What are the characteristics of community medical groups and practitioners that participate actively in clinical research?
- What approaches to enlisting practitioner participation are most successful?
- What approaches to securing trial enrollment and participant retention are most successful in the community practice setting?
- How have community-based research programs succeeded in engaging culturally and linguistically diverse populations?
- How can participation in clinical trials be successfully extended into chronic disease care settings?
- How can clinical trials be organized to maximize practitioner participation?
- What are successful methods of achieving public engagement?
- How have systems, hospitals, and medical groups that are engaged in research developed the necessary workforce competencies?

Summary

The United States faces a pressing need for a revitalized clinical trials infrastructure. But rather than attempting to optimize clinical trials conduct independently of health care delivery, we recommend that clinical trials and clinical care be integrated into the learning health system. The rapid evolution of integrated health systems provides a natural vehicle for accomplishing this goal, using electronic health records aggregated at the health system level and beyond. The one major exception to this approach should be for intensive biological research that we envision as taking place within a system of Innovator's Labs connected by sophisticated informatics and strategic technology investments. The continuation of standardized control trials in the Traditional Labs and the development of Health Care Delivery Labs embedded within integrated health systems will provide a major improvement in the quantity, quality, and generalizability of clinical trial results (see Figure 2). Community Engagement Labs will need to be expanded to conduct critical trials outside traditional health care delivery systems. Intense efforts will be needed in order to understand the requirements for an effective national system capable of interdigitating with developing global systems, including efforts focused on workforce development, economic analysis, and concrete operational plans.

The vision described in this paper for the future of clinical research will require improved alignment among patients, payers, and providers with respect to the implications of research and the choices of each stakeholder regarding receiving, funding, or providing specific services. Assuming that such alignment among stakeholders can be attained, the financial incentives to improve care, avoid waste, redundancy, and unnecessary services could result in better health outcomes, moderation of cost increases, and the opportunity for a jointly financed research and development engine to provide for continuous measurement, innovation, and improvement across the health care continuum. Given the fragmented nature of the American payer and provider landscape, a national "clinical research tax" applied to health care premiums could be a potential source of the funds needed to fuel the research and development engine envisioned in the integrated health care and clinical trials enterprise of the future. Some of the savings enabled by continuous quality improvement in health care could also lower the costs of care and premiums paid by patients, or at the least moderate their continued increase.

The authors developed this paper in the context of the IOM Forum on Drug Discovery, Development, and Translation's 2-year effort to assess the current status of the clinical trials enterprise and to put forward a plan to assure a robust and optimal future for clinical research. The consequences of the problems in the extant system are clear and the need to address them is urgent. There is a compelling opportunity to effectively address the gap between the research enterprise and the delivery system in the near future. We suggest attention to the development of a national agent that will bring the stakeholders together and catalyze the essential realignment of organizational mission and system-wide incentives.

REFERENCES

Behrman R. E., Benner J. S., Brown J. S., McClellan M., Woodcock J., and R. Platt. 2011. Developing the Sentinel System—a national resource for evidence development. *N Engl J Med* 10;364(6):498-499.

Bennet C. L., Silver S. M., Djulbegovic B., et al. 2008. Venous thromboembolism and mortality associated with recombinant erythropoietin and darbepoetin administration for the treatment of cancer-associated anemia. *JAMA* 299:914-924.

Bollyky T. J. 2011. *Safer, Faster, Cheaper: Improving Clinical Trials and Regulatory Pathways to Fight Neglected Diseases: Report of the Center for Global Development Working Group on Clinical Trials and Regulatory Pathways.* Washington, DC: Center for Global Development. http://www.cgdev.org/files/1425588_file_Bollyky_Clinical_Trials_FINAL.pdf (accessed April 11, 2012).

Califf R. M. 2009. Clinical research sites—the underappreciated component of the clinical research system. *JAMA* 302(18):2025-2027.

Califf R. M. and R. A. Harrington. 2011. American industry and the U.S. cardiovascular clinical research enterprise: An appropriate analogy? *J Am Coll Cardiol* 58(7):677-680.

Califf R. M., Zarin D. A., Kramer J. M., Sherman R. E., Aberle L. H., and A. Tasneem. The clinical trials enterprise in the United States as revealed by the development of ClinicalTrials.gov as an integrated database. (In review).

Canadian Institutes of Health Research. 2011. *Annual Report 2010-2011.* http://www.cihr-irsc.gc.ca/e/44144.html (accessed October 18, 2011).

Clinical and Translational Science Awards (CTSAs). 2011. http://www.ctsaweb.org/index.cfm?fuseaction=home.aboutHome (accessed September 27, 2011).

Collins F. S. 2011. *The NIH National Center for Advancing Translational Sciences: How Will It Work?* https://www.dtmi.duke.edu/website-administration/files/Collins%20NCATS%20slides.pdf (accessed September 27, 2011).

Coronary Drug Project Research Group. 1973. The Coronary Drug Project: Design, methods, and baseline results. *Circulation* 47(Suppl 1):11-179.

DeVol R. C., Bedroussian A., and B. Yeo. 2011. The global biomedical industry: Preserving U.S. leadership. *The Milken Institute.* http://www.milkeninstitute.org/publications/publications.taf?function=detail&ID=38801285&cat=resrep (accessed October 18, 2011).

Dzau V. J., Ackerly D. C., Sutton-Wallace P., Merson M. H., Williams R. S., Krishnan K. R., Taber R. C., and R. M. Califf. 2010. The role of academic health science systems in the transformation of medicine. *Lancet* 375(9718):949-953.

Eisenstein E. L., Collins R., Cracknell B. S., et al. 2008. Sensible approaches for reducing clinical trial costs. *Clin Trials* 5(1):75-84.

FasterCures. 2005. *Think Research: Using Electronic Medical Records to Bridge Patient Care and Research. White Paper.* http://www.fastercures.org/objects/pdfs/white_papers/emr_whitepaper.pdf (accessed October 17, 2011).

FDA (Food and Drug Administration). 2006. *Promoting Safe and Effective Drugs for 100 Years.* http://www.fda.gov/AboutFDA/WhatWeDo/History/CentennialofFDA/CentennialEditionof FDAConsumer/ucm093787.htm (accessed September 28, 2011).

FDA. 2007. *Public Law 110-85. The Food and Drug Administration Amendments Act of 2007.* http://www.fda.gov/RegulatoryInformation/Legislation/FederalFoodDrugandCosmeticAct FDCAct/SignificantAmendmentstotheFDCAct/FoodandDrugAdministrationAmendmentsActof2007/FullTextofFDAAALaw/default.htm (accessed May 31, 2011).

FDA. 2011. *FDA Drug Safety Communication: Modified Dosing Recommendations to Improve the Safe Use of Erythropoiesis-Stimulating Agents (ESAs) in Chronic Kidney Disease.* http://www.fda.gov/Drugs/DrugSafety/ucm259639.htm (accessed October 19, 2011).

Fisher R. A. 1926. The arrangement of field experiments. *J Min Agric G Br* 33:503-513.

Getz K. A. 2005. Number of active investigators in FDA-regulated clinical trials drop. *Tufts Center for the Study of Drug Development CSDD Impact Report* 7:1-4.

Getz K. A. 2011. *Public Confidence and Trust Today: A Review of Public Opinion Polls.* http://www.ciscrp.org/downloads/articles/Getz_publicopinion.pdf (accessed October 18, 2011).

Glickman S. W., McHutchison J. G., Peterson E. D., Cairns C. B., Harrington R. A., Califf R. M., and K. A. Schulman. 2009. Ethical and scientific implications of the globalization of clinical research. *N Engl J Med* 360(8):816-823.

Gupta Y. K. and B. M. Padhy. 2011. India's growing participation in global clinical trials. *Trends Pharmacol Sci.* 32(6):327-329.

Hulley S., Grady D., Bush T., et al. 1998. Randomized trial of estrogen plus progestin for secondary prevention of coronary heart disease in postmenopausal women: Heart and Estrogen/progestin Replacement Study (HERS) Research Group. *JAMA* 280:605-613.

Institute of Medicine (IOM). 1995. *Health Services Research: Work force and Educational Issues.* Washington, DC: National Academy Press.

IOM. 2007. *The Learning Healthcare System: Workshop Summary.* Washington, DC: The National Academies Press.

IOM. 2008. *Evidence-Based Medicine and the Changing Nature of Health Care: 2007 IOM Annual Meeting Summary.* Washington, DC: The National Academies Press.

IOM. 2011a. *Engineering a Learning Healthcare System: A Look at the Future: Workshop Summary.* Washington, DC: The National Academies Press.

IOM. 2011b. *Public Engagement and Clinical Trials: New Models and Disruptive Technologies: Workshop Summary.* Washington, DC: The National Academies Press.

Jia H. 2005. China beckons to clinical trial sponsors. *Nat Biotechnol.* 23(7):768.

Kim E. S., Carrigan T. P., and V. Menon. 2011. International participation in cardiovascular randomized controlled trials sponsored by the NHLBI. *J Am Coll Cardiol* (in press).

Kottke T. E., Solberg L. I., Nelson A. F., et al. 2008. Optimizing practice through research: A new perspective to solve an old problem. *Ann Fam Med* 6(5):459-462.

Lee D. H., Vielemeyer O. 2011. Analysis of overall level of evidence behind Infectious Diseases Society of America practice guidelines. *Ann Intern Med* 171:18-22.

Lind J. 1753. *A Treatise on the Scurvy in Three Parts, Containing an Inquiry into the Nature, Causes, and Cure, of That Disease.* http://www.jameslindlibrary.org/illustrating/records/a-treatise-of-the-scurvy-in-three-parts-containing-an-inquiry/title_pages (accessed September 27, 2011).

Mahaffey K. W., Wojdyla D. M., Carroll K., et al. 2011. Ticagrelor compared with clopidogrel by geographic region in the Platelet Inhibition and Patient Outcomes (PLATO) trial. *Circulation* 124(5):544-554.

Medical Research Council. 1948. Streptomycin treatment of pulmonary tuberculosis: A Medical Research Council investigation. *British Medical Journal* 1948(ii):7692.

National Institutes of Health (NIH). 2007. *Understanding Clinical Trials.* http://ClinicalTrials.gov/ct2/info/understand#Q01 (accessed October 19, 2011).

O'Connor C. M., Fiuzat M., Swedberg K., et al. 2011. Influence of global region on outcomes in heart failure β-blocker trials. *J Am Coll Cardiol* 58(9):915-922.

Pfeffer M. A., Burdmann E. A., Chen C. Y., et al. 2009. A trial of darbepoetin alfa in type 2 diabetes and chronic kidney disease. *N Engl J Med* 361:2019-2032.

Pratt C. M. and L. Moye. 1990. The Cardiac Arrhythmia Suppression Trial: Implications for anti-arrhythmic drug development. *J Clin Pharmacol* 30:967-974.

Rossouw J. E., Anderson G. L., Prentice R. L., et al. 2002. Writing Group for the Women's Health Initiative Investigators. Risks and benefits of estrogen plus progestin in healthy postmenopausal women: Principal results from the Women's Health Initiative randomized controlled trial. *JAMA* 288(3):321-333.

Simes R. J., O'Connell R. L., Aylward P. E., et al. 2010. Unexplained international differences in clinical outcomes after acute myocardial infarction and fibrinolytic therapy: Lessons from the Hirulog and Early Reperfusion or Occlusion (HERO)-2 trial. *Am Heart J* 159(6):988-997.

Singh A. K., Szczech L., Tang K. L., et al. 2006. Correction of anemia with epoetin alfa in chronic kidney disease. *N Engl J Med* 355:2085-2098.

The Academy of Medical Sciences. 2011. *A new pathway for the regulation and governance of health research.* http://www.acmedsci.ac.uk/p47prid88.html (accessed September 28, 2011).

Tricoci P., Allen J. M., Kramer J. M., Califf R. M., and S. C. Smith Jr. 2009. Scientific evidence underlying the ACC/AHA clinical practice guidelines. *JAMA* 301:831-841.

Tunis S. R., Benner J., and M. McClellan. 2010. Comparative effectiveness research: Policy context, methods development and research infrastructure. *Stat Med* 30;29(19):1963-1976.

U.S. Census Bureau. 2008. *Projections of the population by selected age groups and sex for the United States: 2010 to 2050 (2008 projections).* http://www.census.gov/population/www/projections/summarytables.html (accessed September 27, 2011).

Yusuf S., Bosch J., Devereaux P. J., et al. 2008. Sensible guidelines for the conduct of large randomized trials. *Clin Trials* 5(1):38-39. Erratum in: *Clin Trials* 2008;5(3):283.

Zerhouni E. A. 2003. The NIH Roadmap. *Science* 302(5642):63-72.

TABLE 1 Characteristics of the Clinical Trials Enterprise, as Seen in the ClinicalTrials.gov Registry

	All Studies	All Interventional Trials	Interventional Trials, 2007-2010
Primary purpose, n/N (%)			
Treatment	59,200/75,778 (78.1)	59,200/75,198 (78.7)	28,605/38,199 (74.9)
Prevention	8,092/75,778 (10.7)	8,092/75,198 (10.8)	4,152/38,199 (10.9)
Diagnostic	2,655/75,778 (3.5)	2,655/75,198 (3.5)	1,489/38,199 (3.9)
Supportive care	1,847/75,778 (2.4)	1,847/75,198 (2.5)	1,290/38,199 (3.4)
Screening	866/75,778 (1.1)	286/75,198 (0.4)	195/38,199 (0.5)
Health services research	900/75,778 (1.2)	900/75,198 (1.2)	733/38,199 (1.9)
Basic science	1,882/75,778 (2.5)	1,882/75,198 (2.5)	1,735/38,199 (4.5)
Educational/counseling/ training	336/75,778 (0.4)	336/75,198 (0.4)	—
Primary purpose missing	20,568/96,346 (21.3)	4,215/79,413 (5.3)	2,771/40,970 (6.8)
Type of intervention, n/N (%)			
Drug	53,441/84,614 (63.2)	52,162/79,410 (65.7)	24,751/40,970 (60.4)
Procedural	10,911/84,614 (12.9)	9,635/79,410 (12.1)	4,104/40,970 (10.0)
Biological	6,841/84,614 (8.1)	6,657/79,410 (8.4)	2,948/40,970 (7.2)
Behavioral	7,134/84,614 (8.4)	6,582/79,410 (8.3)	3,307/40,970 (8.1)
Device	6,662/84,614 (7.9)	6,012/79,410 (7.6)	3,799/40,970 (9.3)
Radiation	2,361/84,614 (2.8)	2,292/79,410 (2.9)	928/40,970 (2.3)
Dietary supplement	2,067/84,614 (2.4)	2,036/79,410 (2.6)	1,603/40,970 (3.9)
Genetic	1,096/84,614 (1.3)	712/79,410 (0.9)	381/40,970 (0.9)
Other	8,211/84,614 (9.7)	6,625/79,410 (8.3)	5,110/40,970 (12.5)

continued

TABLE 1 Continued

	All Studies	All Interventional Trials	Interventional Trials, 2007-2010
Enrollment type, n/N (%)			
Actual, n/N (%)	24,317/75,420 (32.2)	21,282/62,479 (34.1)	11,747/40,214 (29.2)
1-100	13,803/24,111 (57.2)	12,341/21,127 (58.4)	7,566/11,671 (64.8)
101-1,000	8,844/24,111 (36.7)	7,767/21,127 (36.8)	3,744/11,671 (32.1)
1,001-5,000	1,220/24,111 (5.1)	883/21,127 (4.2)	316/11,671 (2.7)
>5,000	244/24,111 (1.0)	136/21,127 (0.6)	45/11,671 (0.4)
Anticipated, n/N (%)	51,103/75,420 (67.8)	41,197/62,479 (65.9)	28,467/40,214 (70.8)
1-100	29,510/51,066 (57.8)	25,405/41,177 (61.7)	17,726/28,458 (62.3)
101-1,000	18,252/51,066 (35.7)	13,997/41,177 (34.0)	9,629/28,458 (33.8)
1,001-5,000	2,536/51,066 (5.0)	1,467/41,177 (3.6)	916/28,458 (3.2)
>5,000	768/51,066 (1.5)	308/41,177 (0.7)	187/28,458 (0.7)
Missing enrollment type	20,926/96,346 (21.7)	16,934/79,413 (21.3)	756/40,970 (1.8)
Lead sponsor classification, n/N (%)			
Industry	31,173/93,436 (32.4)	28,264/79,413 (35.6)	15,248/40,970 (37.2)
NIH	9,215/93,436 (9.6)	5,878/79,413 (7.4)	1,106/40,970 (2.7)
U.S. federal (non-NIH)	1,715/93,436 (1.8)	1,473/79,413 (1.9)	547/40,970 (1.3)
Other	54,243/93,436 (56.3)	43,798/79,413 (55.2)	24,069/40,970 (58.7)

SOURCE: Data extracted from the database for Aggregate Analysis of ClinicalTrials.gov (AACT): https://www.trialstransformation.org/projects/improving-the-public-interface-for-use-of-aggregate-data-in-ClinicalTrials.gov/aact-database-for-aggregate-analysis-of-ClinicalTrials.gov.

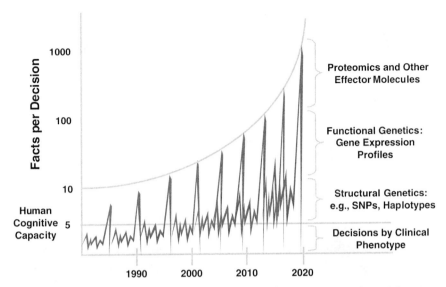

FIGURE 1 Schematic depicting the increase in number of facts per clinical decision with new sources of biological data—that is, the increasing complexity of medical decision making that accompanies biomedical advances.

NOTE: SNP, single-nucleotide polymorphism.

SOURCE: Stead, W. W. 2010. *Recalibrating Informatic's "True North."* Speaker presentation at AMIA Now! 2010, May 27, Phoenix, AZ. http://informatics.mc.vanderbilt. edu/sites/informatics. mc.vanderbilt.edu/files/Stead-AMIA2010-Presentation.pdf (accessed January 6, 2012). Reprinted with permission from William W. Stead.

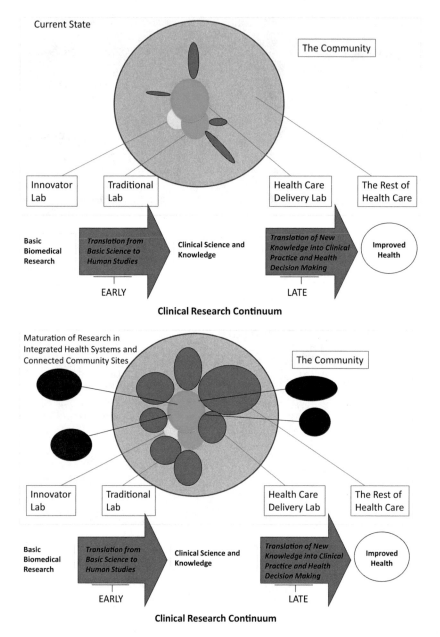

FIGURE 2 This figure depicts the current segmentation of clinical trials enterprise in the United States (top graphic) contrasted with the authors' vision of the potential future organization of clinical trials (bottom graphic) built around the maturation of research in integrated health systems (IHSs) and community sites. Arrows below each figure depict the clinical research continuum from basic research to

improved health. Blue circles indicate IHS-connected community research labs (the fourth type of lab described in this paper). These labs grow in size but stay small in number through mergers and acquisitions in the health system sector. At the same time, community engagement labs not affiliated with an IHS, shown in brown, would be connected to core traditional labs shown in green. These community labs would become larger and more common. Some are all-encompassing, such as the entire city of Rochester, New York.

SOURCE: Adapted from: Sung, N. S. et al. 2003. Central challenges facing the national clinical research enterprise. *JAMA* 289:1278-1287.

Appendix E

Discussion Paper[1]

Developing a Robust Clinical Trials Workforce

Ann Bonham, Association of American Medical Colleges; Robert Califf, Duke Translational Medicine Institute; Elaine Gallin, QE Philanthropic Advisors; and Michael Lauer, National Heart, Lung, and Blood Institute[2]

INTRODUCTION

The gap between the growing demand for evidence to inform practice and our current state of knowledge calls for serious consideration about the best approach to developing a workforce capable of meeting those demands. As referenced in the discussion paper *The Clinical Trials Enterprise in the United States: A Call for Disruptive Innovation* (Califf et al., 2012), the clinical trials enterprise (CTE) is falling behind in the need for evidence, especially in the United States. We envision a need for a clinical research workforce organized in several dimensions that reflect the broad missions of the CTE, the specific disciplines involved, and the level of desirable expertise. The latter could range from broad participation in the CTE to expert participation, and to conceptualization and research on the methods employed by the CTE.

In addition, this workforce must be broadened tremendously to meet the goal implicit in the creation of a true learning health system: the inte-

[1] The views expressed in this discussion paper are those of the authors and not necessarily of the authors' organizations or of the Institute of Medicine. The paper is intended to help inform and stimulate discussion. It has not been subjected to the review procedures of the Institute of Medicine and is not a report of the Institute of Medicine or of the National Research Council.

[2] Participants in the activities of the IOM Forum on Drug Discovery, Development, and Translation. This discussion paper was presented in draft form at the Forum's November 2011 workshop, Envisioning a Transformed Clinical Trials Enterprise in the United States: Establishing an Agenda for 2020, and finalized by the authors following the workshop.

gration of research and continuous learning into practice. However, the more traditional arenas of mechanistic research and efficacy trials call for specialized workforces that until now have all too often depended on ad hoc, "on-the-job" learning, as opposed to the prospective training and education that defines a mature discipline. Finally, the new field of community engagement requires special skills that blend traditional clinical trials knowledge with social and organizational constructs.

The challenge is considerable, because most roles in clinical research at their core involve human experimentation and require specific expertise in a clinical or scientific discipline. Moreover, this expertise must be augmented by focused training in the standards and principles that undergird the conduct of particular types of clinical trials, which range from small, intensive mechanistic studies to very large, community-based interventions.

A Salutary Example: The Occluded Artery Trial (OAT)

One example of the need for broadening the discipline to include medical practitioners is the recent OAT Trial, a cardiology study funded by the National Institutes of Health (NIH). In the 1990s, cardiologists sought to understand how best to manage patients who survived the first few days of ST-segment-elevation acute myocardial infarction (STEMI), but with persistent total occlusions of their infarct-related artery. The enormous benefits of rapid reperfusion in the acute phase of STEMI had already been established in well-controlled clinical trials. Although the detection of an occluded artery several days after the onset of the STEMI would come too late for treatment to be effective in salvaging damaged heart muscle, cardiologists wondered whether there might still be benefit in deploying stents to open up the occluded arteries; the newly opened arteries might supply blood to "watershed" areas at the edge of the infarct zone, thereby reducing the risk of life-threatening arrhythmias and other major events. Further, experimental evidence suggested that the infarction might heal more effectively with perfusion.

Some investigators analyzed observational cohorts and found that patients who were discharged with patent arteries did indeed fare better. The "open artery hypothesis" was alive and supported by observational evidence, so much so that for many cardiologists it became standard practice to ensure that their STEMI patients went home with an open artery.

However, some academic cardiologists questioned whether routine post-STEMI stenting of persistently occluded arteries was of clinical value: Did this practice actually improve clinical outcomes? With support from the National Heart, Lung, and Blood Institute (NHLBI), they organized OAT, a multicenter clinical trial in which patients would be randomly assigned to optimal medical therapy alone or to optimal medical therapy combined with stent placement.

Although STEMI is hardly a rare condition, the investigators experienced enormous difficulty enrolling patients. Most of the American hospitals they approached refused to participate, because domestic cardiologists were convinced of the value of routine post-STEMI stenting. By the time the trial was complete, nearly three-quarters of the study participants enrolled were from research sites outside the United States.

And the results of OAT were surprising. Contrary to expectations, patients who were randomly assigned to stenting seemed to fare slightly worse than those assigned to medical therapy alone. The results, which were published in the *New England Journal of Medicine* (Hochman, 2006), led to rapid changes in cardiology practice guidelines. Yet, 5 years after the OAT study was published, there has been little change in practice. Many cardiologists continue to routinely deploy stents in stable post-infarct STEMI patients, despite the absence of evidence of benefit (and despite the evidence of absence of benefit), and in direct contradiction to the clear recommendations of their own professional societies.

The OAT experience encapsulates what is wrong with how clinical trials are perceived, implemented, and interpreted in the United States. Relatively few U.S. patients participated, in large part because their American cardiologists were not engaged. As was discussed at a 2009 Institute of Medicine (IOM) workshop, OAT also highlighted misaligned financial incentives because physicians are focused on performing a high volume of procedures, which creates a disincentive for them to refer patients to a clinical trial to receive a procedure (IOM, 2009). Also, the lengthy timeline to conduct a large, multicenter trial hinders medical learning and potential benefits to patients. The OAT trial took 10 years from hypothesis generation to completion. Even though the trial has been completed and its results communicated, many American patients are not benefitting from the findings, because their cardiologists have not changed their practices. Nor is the OAT experience unique or even unusual; the difficulty experienced across fields by American clinical trialists seeking to enroll patients and engage practitioners is well documented.

Clinical Research: A Public Good?

Two years ago, Schaefer, Emanuel, and Wertheimer (Schaefer et al., 2009) argued for a "cultural shift in the moral framework that is brought to participation in research." They suggested that clinical research should be regarded as a "public good" in which all people stand to benefit, whether they actively participate or not. But if research is a public good, people should then aim to participate in research unless there is a compelling reason not to, "participation being a moral obligation for everyone to do his part."

Such a view may seem extreme. Should we go so far as to expect, not just encourage, participation in research? But, in fact, evidence suggests that the majority of Americans would be willing to participate if asked. However, only 7 percent of American adults say that their doctors have ever suggested that they participate in a clinical study (Charlton Research Company, 2007). In one study of specialty physicians, one-third of physicians affiliated with an organization designed to support clinical trial participation were not actively engaged in the research process (Klabunde et al., 2011). In other words, many Americans would gladly participate, but their doctors aren't asking.

Some commentators have lamented that American doctors seem to have little interest in science as a way to drive their practices. Even doctors' professional societies, which have some degree of scientific orientation, routinely issue guidelines of which only a small proportion are based on evidence from high-quality randomized trials, a point reinforced by recent publications examining guidelines for cardiology (Tricoci et al., 2009) and infectious diseases (Lee and Vielemeyer, 2011). Thus, the paucity of physician and public engagement cannot be ascribed to our knowing all the answers—we aren't even a fraction of the way there.

In our view, the largest segment of the clinical trials workforce comprises all individuals—the general public—including the diverse communities and neighborhoods across the United States. Individuals should not only participate in trials as volunteers but should be viewed as partners in the clinical trials enterprise with the ability to mobilize their friends, families, and communities to drive change. This segment of the workforce has the important responsibility of working in partnership with clinicians to identify the important questions about care that need answers through a clinical trial. The future of research might also be headed in the direction of e-trials, where there are no investigative sites or physicians/middlemen. Individuals with a smart phone or a computer can enroll in an e-trial directly through a website. In this sense, individual patients could truly become the largest segment of the clinical trials workforce. In terms of training, the public should be educated as to the value of clinical research and the link between clinical trials and improvements in care. This broad-based appreciation and understanding of the value of clinical research could be instilled via national public service announcements, key opinion leaders and policy makers, and the greater integration of science education, and specifically clinical research, in K-12 programs.

In partnership with the public, the next largest segment of the clinical trials workforce would be, in some respects, no different from the clinical care workforce. In a true learning health system, every patient with an incurable disease—and that is eventually most of us—would present an opportunity for active learning. Each practicing clinician and his or her consenting patients would be engaged in a massive tapestry of well-designed trials that would enable all of us to answer real-world questions in the most robust way possible: through randomization.

Some have argued that routine implementation of electronic health records (EHRs) and large-scale registries would suffice. While these tools would make observational research easier, they cannot by themselves enable rigorous scientific evaluation of the most important clinical questions, which can only be properly addressed with randomization.

We view the ideal clinical trials workforce as one in which all clinicians think scientifically. When confronted with a clinical problem for which definitive evidence is lacking, the clinician's first thought should be, "What good trial would apply here? How can my patient and I be part of the solution?" Of course, effective deployment of EHRs with standardized data elements would allow randomized controlled trials (RCTs) to be done at a much lower cost by reducing or eliminating redundant data collection, but unless knowledge generation is embraced as a fundamental component of practice, the gap between existing evidence and practice needs will remain cavernous.

The ideal clinical trials workforce will be orders of magnitude larger than its present size, because it will include nearly all of the 90 percent of clinicians who currently are not part of the clinical trials enterprise. These clinicians will embrace research as a critical, indeed morally imperative, component of their work as medical professionals. They will work closely with professional clinical trialists who implement clinical research in the context of practice and will collaborate with them to prioritize, design, analyze, and interpret the trials that will be embedded into their practices. Of course, with a much larger proportion of American clinical practitioners and patients participating in the trials, there will also be an acute need for a larger workforce of professional trialists and clinical research professionals (see Table 1: Core Competencies in Clinical and Translational Research).

COMPETENCIES, FUNCTION, AND LOCUS OF NEEDED WORKFORCE

Realizing the vision of a significantly expanded clinical trials workforce will require major training efforts, both for new and veteran health care workers. A core set of competencies, including principles of responsible trials conduct and the fundamentals of study design, should be part of training programs for most of the clinical trials and clinical care workforce,[3] although the level of information provided would vary depending on workers' backgrounds and responsibilities. However, while identifying core competencies may result in a better-informed workforce, the complex nature of the CTE precludes a "one-size-fits-all" training program. Developing a highly competent workforce will require instruction in two additional dimensions—discipline- and job-specific training and education. In the team-based CTE (and, for that matter, clinical care) environment of the future, training in teamwork and understanding across disciplines will be needed. Facts can be learned interchangeably by experts in different areas, but fundamental knowledge must be transmitted in an effective manner.

Dimension 1: Defining the Workforce

In order to simplify this discussion, we have parsed the clinical trials workforce of the future into five groups, beginning with a very broad-based group and progressing to smaller, more focused workforce groups (see Figure 1 for a schematic of the workforce groups):

- **Group 1:** Individuals from the community who understand, support, and participate in clinical trials (referred to as *the public*)
- **Group 2:** The clinical workforce who participate in trials as part of their clinical practices (referred to as *community practitioners*)
- **Group 3:** Clinical trialists who devote specified portions of their professional efforts to serving as principal investigators or collaborating co-investigators at clinical research sites, with primary responsibility for implementing clinical trials at the level of a hospital or research site (referred to as *implementers*)
- **Group 4:** Investigators who lead and design clinical trials, as well as scientific experts who develop tools and innovative approaches for conducting trials (referred to as *investigators*)
- **Group 5:** Academicians who explore the methodologies of conducting clinical trials (referred to as *methodologists*).

---

[3] "NCATS [National Center for Advancing Translational Sciences], in collaboration with the CTSA [Clinical and Translational Science Awards] Education and Career Development Key Function Committee, formed the Education Core Competency Work Group to define the training standards for core competencies in clinical and translational research. The work group's final recommendations for core competencies include 14 thematic areas that should shape the training experiences of junior investigators by defining the skills, attributes, and knowledge that can be shared across multidisciplinary teams of clinician-scientists" (https://www.ctsacentral.org/committee/education-and-career-development).

The middle groups—*investigators* and *implementers*—will have many overlapping areas of competence, but the level of training (doctoral- versus masters-level training) and scope of the discipline-specific expertise needed to carry out their work is expected to be less for implementers than for investigators (who design and lead trials), or for methodologists (who develop new approaches to the design, conduct, or analysis of trials). Nonetheless, the workforce falling within either of these two groups must be expanded considerably if the promise of universal participation in clinical trials leading to a health system founded on evidence-based medicine is to be met.

The sections below outline the required training, responsibilities, and locations in which the groups work.

Group 1: The Public. This workforce group comprises the nation as a whole and includes all individuals in communities across the country. Individuals consider research a public good and participate in studies unless they have a compelling reason not to do so. Educating the public and inspiring the concept of research as a public good requires strong national leadership.

Group 2: Community Practitioners. This group comprises *practitioners* who participate in trials as part of their clinical practice. Community practitioners include primary caregivers (physicians, nurses, pharmacists, etc.) and social service employees working at the community level. Their training needs to include an introduction to clinical trials as well as some of the core competencies in translational and clinical research, as defined by many of the Clinical and Translational Science Awards (CTSA) programs (see Table 1: CTSA Core Competencies, p. 13). However, if CTSA-like training materials are used, they will in some cases need to be simplified to align with the skill-set of the targeted workforce. These workers are typically found where primary and secondary health care are delivered.

Group 3: Implementers. This group is primarily responsible for implementing clinical trials at the level of a hospital or research site. Implementers will include physician-scientists, nurse-investigators, operations specialists, data managers, computer specialists, pharmacists, social service personnel, and others vital to the implementation of clinical trials. A major part of the implementation workforce will include clinical research coordinators (CRCs) and professional research-site managers (RSMs) working within academic centers, contract research organizations, industry, hospitals, and large clinics.

As with Group 4 described below, Group 3 implementers receive both discipline-specific specialty training and CTSA-style training in core competencies for translational and clinical research. However, the level of the training for these personnel is likely to be more pragmatic (less conceptual) and training will likely require fewer years than that for the investigators in Group 4. For example, pharmacists, nurse-investigators, and data managers making up a clinical trials implementation team do not need to hold doctoral-level degrees, and many of these jobs are currently accomplished by individuals with bachelors-level education coupled with discipline-specific training offered by organizations such as the Association of Clinical Research Professionals (ACRP).

There is a critical need to expand this part of the clinical trials workforce and improve its core competencies. In addition, in order to address the need for recruiting more diverse patient populations and to accommodate the trend toward multinational clinical trials, this workforce expansion needs to include an increase in worker diversity.

Group 4: Investigators. Personnel in this group are charged with leading and designing clinical trials. The rubric "Investigator" also includes scientific experts who develop tools and innovative approaches for conducting trials, and while there is overlap, it is useful to consider investigators of specific projects as different from those who develop new methods (Group 5 below). Investigators comprise MD-, MD/PhD-, and PhD-level investigators from many different disciplines. This highly trained workforce is needed not only to lead and design clinical trials but also to advance the area of "Regulatory Sciences," defined by the Food and Drug Administration (FDA) as "the science of developing new tools, standards and approaches to assess the safety, efficacy, quality, and performance of FDA-regulated products" (FDA, 2011). Advances in regulatory sciences will require personnel with expertise in new technologies, including imaging, cell and tissue engineering, and nanotechnology. In addition, the current major shortage of biostatisticians and informaticists across academic medicine, industry, and government must be addressed.

We expect that most persons falling within this category will need extensive graduate and postgraduate training in discipline-specific areas such as epidemiology, computational biology, and genomics, and/or disease-specific areas such as cardiology and infectious diseases. In addition, the required scientific/clinical discipline-specific training can be supplemented as needed by core training in translational and clinical research offered through the CTSA. In order to effectively leverage scientific opportunities and stimulate innovative approaches, the traditional departmental training silos must be broken down to encourage investigators to train and work across disciplines.

Most investigators currently can be found within academic health science systems (AHSSs), professional research sites, and community practices that conduct research, as well as in the pharmaceutical and medical device industries. A smaller number work at government agencies such as NIH, the Centers for Disease Control and Prevention, and FDA; others work with public–private partnerships such as the Medicines for Malaria Initiative. In the future, more AHSSs will be transforming themselves into integrated systems, enabling the efficient bridging of translational gaps between discovery and health care. Such organizations will require many more highly trained clinical trial investigators.

Group 5: Methodologists. This last group includes experts who perform research on the methods and policies pertinent to clinical trials. This relatively small yet substantial cadre of clinical investigators, biostatisticians, epidemiologists, and health services researchers is vital to advancing clinical trials methods. These experts will be located within AHSSs, government, research institutes, and some large industry groups with capacity to fund protected time for research.

Dimension 2: Critical Disciplines

The second dimension of the workforce is the scientific discipline in which the individual works. Our major thesis is that all health care providers (practitioners) should be trained in the fundamentals of participating in research and should be taught that knowledge generation is a fundamental professional responsibility of health care delivery. This extends not only to physicians and nurses, but also to physician assistants, respiratory therapists, physical therapists, pharmacists, and other providers. Any of these professions can produce either implementers or investigators. Many of the investigators and methodologists will be epidemiologists, biostatisticians, and informaticists.

There is currently a critical shortage of biostatisticians and informaticists across academic medicine, industry, and government. Serious efforts are needed in order to develop this segment of the workforce. The costs of training this critical cadre of the workforce are small compared with the overall research budget of the relevant funding organizations, and a modest investment would have a multiplier effect on the quality of clinical trials.

Dimension 3: Critical Competencies and Special Knowledge

The third dimension is competency and special educational knowledge. In the team-based research environment of the future, much of the material can be learned interchangeably by experts in different areas, but the fundamental knowledge remains to be transmitted in an effective manner.

DEMOGRAPHIC TRENDS INFLUENCING WORKFORCE NEEDS

Demographic trends in diverse and aging populations, and the intersections of these trends with systematic health disparities, are significant factors affecting the development of a robust and diverse workforce that will design, perform, and participate in clinical trials, as well as communicate research findings to all relevant populations.

Demographic Shifts

The U.S. Census Bureau projects 334 million people in the United States by 2020, up from 310 million in 2010 (U.S. Census Bureau, 2009). By 2050, this number is expected to grow to nearly 400 million (assuming net-constant immigration). As is well known, the ethnic composition of the U.S. population is also changing, such that by 2050 no single ethnicity will characterize a majority of Americans. Perhaps the most notable shift will be the number of people identified in the U.S. Census as being of Hispanic origin. This demographic group is expected to increase from a current 16 percent of the population (49 million) to 19 percent (55 million) in 2020, on a trajectory to include one in five Americans (70 million) by 2025. All ethnicities tracked by the census will increase in absolute numbers, although this increase will be to varying degrees considered as a percentage of the population.

White persons not identifying as Hispanic or other ethnicities will increase from 201 million to 204 million, but will decline from 65 percent of the population to 61 percent by 2020. Black or African American non-Hispanic persons will increase from 38 million to 41 million by 2020 (a 9 percent increase) but will remain about 12 percent of the total population over the decade. The fastest growth continues to be among Asians and Native Hawaiian/Pacific Islanders (now classified separately), both growing by more than 20 percent from 2010 to 2020, although remaining under 5 percent and under 1 percent of the general population, respectively.

This changing racial and ethnic composition will also be accompanied by the aging of the U.S. population. As underscored in recent news reports, the first cohort of "Baby Boomers"—the generation of Americans born between 1946 and 1964—reaches 65 years of age this year. The number of Americans 65 and older, now 40 million (13 percent of the U.S. population), will increase correspondingly, reaching 16 percent of the population by 2020 and nearly 20 percent of the total population by 2025. According to the Population Reference Bureau, more than 20 percent of this 65-plus cohort will be grouped with the "oldest old"—persons ages 85 and older. Oldest-old persons will number 19 million by 2050—a number greater than the populations of most U.S. states today (Population Reference Bureau, 2011). This aging of the general population is also largely a global phenomenon, at least for many developed nations. In fact, the U.S. population of persons aged 18 and under will remain nearly stable, decreasing slightly from a current 24.1 percent to 23.8 percent by 2020.

Other notable population factors, although too complex to consider in detail in this discussion, include increasing variations in income distribution in the United States, as reported in recent communications on the increase in the number of Americans living below the federally estimated poverty line. These reports show troubling trends: recent economic stresses have resulted in a 7 percent increase (to 31 million) in the number of children living in low-income families. Childhood poverty may emerge as an increasingly important determinant of clinical research needs in the future.

Health Disparities

The U.S. Department of Health and Human Services (HHS) has defined a *health disparity* as a particular type of health difference that is closely linked with social, economic, and/or environmental disadvantage. As HHS notes:

> Racial and ethnic minorities still lag behind in many health outcome measures. They are less likely to get the preventive care they need to stay healthy, more likely to suffer from serious illnesses, such as diabetes or heart disease, and when they do get sick, are less likely to have access to quality health care. (HHS, 2011)

Disparities identified by HHS relate to infant mortality, asthma, diabetes, flu, cancer, HIV/AIDS, chronic lower-respiratory disease, cardiovascular disease, viral hepatitis, chronic liver disease and cirrhosis, kidney disease, injury deaths, violence, behavioral health, and oral health (HHS, 2011).

The extent of these disparities as a pressing national health issue was recently documented by the IOM (2004), and is the subject of many federal and independent initiatives (AHRQ, 2010), including a 2011 action plan under the Affordable Care Act. One of the plan's five goals is to advance scientific knowledge and innovation relating to health disparities through data collection and promoting patient-centered outcomes research. A second major goal focuses on improvements to workforce development, including through

> a new pipeline program for recruiting undergraduates from underserved communities for public health and biomedical sciences careers, expanding and improving health care interpreting and translation, and supporting more training of community health workers, such as *promotoras*. (HHS, 2011)

Redressing health disparities will require both a more extensive network for clinical trials and a workforce skilled in community engagement. Clinical trials must be crafted to assess the effects of disparities for separate populations, including by age (discussed below)—aspects that could greatly complicate trial design and analysis. In order to gauge the impact of health disparities on different populations and assess which interventions are truly most effective for diverse communities, the national CTE will need to engage in multisite trials covering broad geographic ranges and including many provider organizations. Along with these challenges, there is enormous potential for such research to improve the overall health of the nation, especially where biological mechanisms supporting an intervention in one segment of the population are already well understood, and may be adapted in a straightforward manner to other populations.

The Burden of Disease Related to an Aging Population

The increasing size and proportion of the national population aged 65 years and older (and the growing subset of the population aged 85 years and older) present new considerations related to the burden of disease. In the United States as elsewhere, a disproportionate share of medical services is provided to older populations. We might thus expect that older persons would be the subject of research aimed at providing the best evidence of which therapies work best in the older population. However, Zulman and colleagues have found that one in five trials examined excluded patients because of age, and nearly half of the remainder included criteria that made participation by older subjects less likely. In addition, fewer than 40 percent of trials examined reported results for different subgroups by age. A further complication is that older patients are more likely to have chronic or other conditions unrelated to a trial's topic of study, which results in their exclusion. The combined result of these factors is a shortfall in evidence to inform the optimal treatment of older patients with multiple health conditions (Zulman et al., 2011).

For example, in 2011 an estimated 5.4 million Americans of all ages had Alzheimer's disease, 5.2 million of whom were age 65 or older (Alzheimer's Association, 2011). Without any breakthrough in preventing or treating the disease and as the population of older persons increases, between 11 million and 16 million people age 65 and older are projected to have Alzheimer's disease by 2050. Medicare beneficiaries age 65 and older with Alzheimer's disease and/or other dementias have tripled the average Medicare costs of other beneficiaries. One estimate calculates that in the absence of any new effective treatments, the cumulative costs of care for people with Alzheimer's disease from 2010 to 2050 will exceed

$20 trillion in 2010 dollars (Alzheimer's Association, 2010). The impact of advances from clinical trials in this field alone could have enormous economic consequences, and potentially could single-handedly bend the health care cost curve in a more affordable direction.

Implications for a Clinical Trials Workforce

A diverse, inclusive workforce helps to build trust among diverse research participants through outreach and engagement with communities. A diverse workforce can constitute the foundation for increased participation in research by underrepresented groups, and can even change the nature of the questions addressed by clinical trials.

Such a workforce strengthens the design, conduct, or support of clinical trials. A professional commitment to focusing on particular areas of disease, pursuing particular lines of research, or working with different communities or populations is greatly determined by personal experience. A diversity of backgrounds helps ensure a sufficient range of experiences, interests, and corresponding dedication among investigators to address relevant topics for clinical trials in a population as diverse as the United States'.

This is not to say that investigators and health workers should confine their interests to communities where they live or grew up; in academic settings, it appears to be the norm that clinical investigators and health professionals cross broad cultural, social, and geographic boundaries to conduct their research. But researchers uniformly cite their personal backgrounds, experiences, and early motivations as critical to the later development of their careers and as influential in their choice of the areas of medicine they practice.

A key requirement, which is common to the scientific and medical research enterprise at large, is to ensure that talent and skills are drawn from across all segments of the U.S. population. Despite a record of rapid growth in public and private investment in medical research up to the current decade, despite growing interests from minority and international students in medical and health care fields, and despite many notable instances of accomplishment by prominent minority scientists, academic research has not succeeded in expanding the participation of underrepresented groups, including African Americans and Hispanic or Latino Americans in the research career pipeline. Nor has academic medicine been notably successful in advancing or retaining minority scientists within research careers. There are also notable disparities by gender in recruitment, advancement, and retention of MD or PhD scientists, which in one sense can exacerbate underrepresentation by some minorities for whom women are more likely than men to earn baccalaureate degrees—a preliminary requirement for careers in science. Especially troubling is a recent NIH analysis showing that even well-established minority scientists are 10 percent less likely than other applicants to receive R01 research grants, raising concerns that similar disparities might plague minority scientists in applications for clinical trials (Ginther et al., 2011).

The failure to engage sufficient involvement of minorities in clinical trials is exemplified in FDA's recent approval of belimumab, the first new drug for the treatment of systemic lupus erythematosus to be approved in more than 50 years. In trials, belimumab relieved symptoms of lupus in about 43 perecnt of patients receiving the active drug, compared with 34 percent of those receiving placebo. However, the trial did not demonstrate significant benefit for African Americans, who have a higher incidence of lupus than whites. According to press reports, FDA said that there were "too few African Americans in the trials to draw a definitive conclusion" (Pollack, 2011).

Finally, discussions related to the definition of the clinical trials workforce could prompt examination of the question of "who" is the workforce. Imagine, for instance, a future in which all citizens—including all providers—view themselves as working hand-in-glove with the clinical trials research workforce as part of a collective commitment to improving the health of the nation.

REFERENCES

Agency for Healthcare Research and Quality (AHRQ). 2010. *National Healthcare Disparities Report.* http://www.ahrq.gov/qual/nhdr10/nhdr10.pdf (accessed October 13, 2011).

Alzheimer's Association. 2010. *Changing the Trajectory of Alzheimer's Disease: A National Imperative.* http://www.alz.org/alzheimers_disease_trajectory.asp (accessed October 13, 2011).

Alzheimer's Association. 2011. *2011 Alzheimer's Disease Facts and Figures.* http://www.alz. org/downloads/Facts_Figures_2011.pdf (accessed October 13, 2011).

Califf, R., G. Filerman, R. Murray, and M. Rosenblatt. 2012. *The Clinical Trials Enterprise in the United States: A Call for Disruptive Innovation.* Discussion Paper, Institute of Medicine, Washington, DC. http://www.iom.edu/Global/Perspectives/2012/CallforCTE.aspx (accessed April 23, 2012).

Charlton Research Company. 2007. *A Public Opinion Study for Research!America.* http:// www.researchamerica.org/uploads/poll.report.2007.transforminghealth.pdf (accessed October 12, 2011).

FDA (Food and Drug Administration). 2011. *Advancing Regulatory Sciences at the FDA: Strategic Plan 2011.* http://www.fda.gov/ScienceResearch/SpecialTopics/RegulatoryScience/ucm268095.htm (accessed October 13, 2011).

Ginther D. K., W. T. Schaffer, J. Schnell, B. Masimore, F. Liu, L. Haak, and R. Kington. 2011. Race, ethnicity, and NIH research awards. *Science* 333:1015-1019.

HHS (Department of Health and Human Services). 2011. *HHS Action Plan to Reduce Health Disparities.* http://www.hhs.gov/news/press/2011pres/04/20110408a.html (accessed October 13, 2011).

Hochman, J. S., et al. 2006. Coronary intervention for persistent occlusion after myocardial infarction. *New England Journal of Medicine* 355:2395-2407.

IOM (Institute of Medicine). 2004. *In the Nation's Compelling Interest: Ensuring Diversity in the Health-Care Workforce*. Washington, DC: The National Academies Press.

IOM. 2009. *Transforming Clinical Research in the United States: Challenges and Opportunities: Workshop Summary*. Washington, DC: The National Academies Press.

Klabunde, C. N., N. L. Keating, A. L. Potosky, A. Ambs, Y. He, M. C. Hornbrook, and P. A. Ganz. 2011. A population-based assessment of specialty physician involvement in cancer clinical trials. *Journal of the National Cancer Institute* 103:384-397.

Lee, D. H., and O. Vielemeyer. 2011. Analysis of overall level of evidence behind Infectious Diseases Society of America practice guidelines. *Annals of Internal Medicine* 171:18-22.

Pollack, A. 2011. FDA approves drug for Lupus, an innovation after 50 years. *New York Times*, March 9. http://www.nytimes.com/2011/03/10/health/10drug.html (accessed October 13, 2011).

Population Reference Bureau. 2011. *America's Aging Population*. http://www.prb.org/pdf11/aging-in-america.pdf (accessed October 13, 2011).

Schaefer, G. O., E. J. Emanuel, and A. Wertheimer. 2009. The obligation to participate in biomedical research. *JAMA* 302(1):67-72.

Tricoci P., J. M. Allen, J. M. Kramer, R. M. Califf, and S. C. Smith Jr. 2009. Scientific evidence underlying the ACC/AHA clinical practice guidelines. *JAMA* 301:831-841.

U.S. Census Bureau. 2009. *Table 1-C. Projections of the Population and Components of Change for the United States: 2010 to 2050 Constant Net International Migration Series (NP2009-T1-C)*. http://www.census.gov/population/www/projections/2009cnmsSumTabs.html (accessed October 13, 2011).

Zulman, D. M., J. B. Sussman, X. Chen, C. T. Cigolle, C. S. Blaum, and R. A. Hayward. 2011. Examining the evidence: A systematic review of the inclusion and analysis of older adults in randomized controlled trials. *Journal of General Internal Medicine* 26(7):783-790.

TABLE 1 Core Competencies in Clinical and Translational Research from the CTSA Education and Career Development Committee, Education Core Competency Work Group

Core Thematic Areas	Competencies
I. Clinical & translational research questions	• Identify basic and preclinical studies that are potential testable clinical research hypotheses. • Identify research observations that could be the bases of large clinical trials. • Define the data that formulate research hypotheses. • Derive translational questions from clinical research data. • Prepare the background and significance sections of a research proposal. • Critique clinical and translational research questions using data-based literature searches. • Extract information from the scientific literature that yields scientific insight for research innovation.
II. Literature critique	• Conduct a comprehensive and systematic search of the literature using informatics techniques. • Summarize evidence from the literature on a clinical problem. • Describe the mechanism of a clinical problem reviewed in a manuscript. • Use evidence as the basis of the critique and interpretation of results of published studies. • Identify potential sources of bias and variations in published studies. • Interpret published literature in a causal framework. • Identify gaps in knowledge within a research problem.
III. Study design	• Formulate a well-defined clinical or translational research question to be studied in human or animal models. • Propose study designs for addressing a clinical or translational research question. • Assess the strengths and weaknesses of possible study designs for a given clinical or translational research question. • Design a research study protocol. • Identify a target population for a clinical or translational research project. • Identify measures to be applied to a clinical or translational research project. • Design a research data analysis plan. • Determine resources needed to implement a clinical or translational research plan. • Prepare an application to an institutional review board (IRB).

continued

TABLE 1 Continued

Core Thematic Areas	Competencies
IV. Research implementation	• Compare the feasibility, efficiency, and ability to derive unbiased inferences from different clinical and translational research study designs. • Assess threats to internal validity in any planned or completed clinical or translational study, including selection bias, misclassification, and confounding. • Incorporate regulatory precepts into the design of any clinical or translational study. • Integrate elements of translational research into given study designs that could provide the bases for future research, such as the collection of biological specimens nested studies and the development of community-based interventions.
V. Sources of error	• Describe the concepts and implications of reliability and validity of study measurements. • Evaluate the reliability and validity of measures. • Assess threats to study validity (bias) including problems with sampling, recruitment, randomization, and comparability of study groups. • Differentiate between the analytic problems that can be addressed with standard methods and those requiring input from biostatisticians and other scientific experts. • Implement quality-assurance systems with control procedures for data intake, management, and monitoring for different study designs. • Assess data sources and data quality to answer specific clinical or translational research questions. • Implement quality-assurance and quality-control procedures for different study designs and analysis.

continued

TABLE 1 Continued

Core Thematic Areas	Competencies
VI. Statistical approaches	• Describe the role that biostatistics serves in biomedical and public health research. • Describe the basic principles and practical importance of random variation, systematic error, sampling error, measurement error, hypothesis testing, type I and type II errors, and confidence limits. • Scrutinize the assumptions behind different statistical methods and their corresponding limitations. • Generate simple descriptive and inferential statistics that fit the study design chosen and answer research question. • Compute sample size, power, and precision for comparisons of two independent samples with respect to continuous and binary outcomes. • Describe the uses of meta-analytic methods. • Defend the significance of data- and safety-monitoring plans. • Collaborate with biostatisticians in the design, conduct, and analyses of clinical and translational research. • Evaluate computer output containing the results of statistical procedures and graphics. • Explain the uses, importance, and limitations of early stopping rules in clinical trials.
VII. Biomedical informatics	• Describe trends and best practices in informatics for the organization of biomedical and health information. • Develop protocols utilizing management of information using computer technology. • Describe the effects of technology on medical research, education, and patient care. • Describe the essential functions of the EHR and the barriers to its use. • Explain the role that health information technology (IT) standards have on the interoperability of clinical systems, including health IT messaging. • Access patient information using quality checks via EHR systems. • Retrieve medical knowledge through literature searches using advanced electronic techniques. • Discuss the role of bioinformatics in the study design and analyses of high-dimensional data in areas such as genotypic and phenotypic genomics. • Collaborate with bioinformatics specialists in the design, development, and implementation of research projects.

continued

TABLE 1 Continued

Core Thematic Areas	Competencies
VIII. Responsible conduct of research	*VIII.a. Clinical Research Ethics Competencies* • Summarize the history of research abuses and the rationale for creating codes, regulations, and systems for protecting participants in clinical research that requires community input. • Critique a clinical or translational research proposal for risks to human subjects. • Explain the special issues that arise in research with vulnerable participants and the need for additional safeguards. • Determine the need for a risk-benefit ratio that is in balance with the outcomes in clinical and translational research. • Describe the elements of voluntary informed consent, including increasing knowledge about research, avoiding undue influence or coercion, and assuring the decision-making capacity of participants. • Assure the need for privacy protection throughout all phases of a study. • Assure the need for fairness in recruiting participants and in distributing the benefits and burdens of clinical research. • Adhere to IRB application procedures. • Explain how the structural arrangement of science and the research industry may influence the behavior of scientists and the production of scientific knowledge. *VIII.b. Responsible Conduct of Research Competencies* • Apply the main rules, guidelines, codes, and professional standards for the conduct of clinical and translational research. • Adhere to the procedures to report unprofessional behavior by colleagues who engage in misconduct in research. • Implement procedures for the identification, prevention, and management of financial, intellectual, and employment conflicts of interest. • Apply the rules and professional standards that govern data collection, sharing, and protection throughout all phases of clinical and translational research. • Apply elements of voluntary informed consent, of fostering understanding of information about clinical research, and for avoiding undue influence or coercion, and taking into consideration the decision-making capacity of participants. • Explain the need for privacy protection and best practices for protecting privacy throughout all phases of a study. • Explain the need for fairness in recruiting participants and in distributing the benefits and burdens of clinical research. • Explain the function of the IRB.

continued

TABLE 1 Continued

Core Thematic Areas	Competencies
IX. Scientific communication	• Communicate clinical and translational research findings to different groups of individuals, including colleagues, students, the lay public, and the media. • Translate the implications of clinical and translational research findings for clinical practice, advocacy, and governmental groups. • Write summaries of scientific information for use in the development of clinical health care policy. • Translate clinical and translational research findings into national health strategies or guidelines for use by the general public. • Explain the utility and mechanism of commercialization for clinical and translational research findings, the patent process, and technology transfer.
X. Cultural diversity	• Differentiate between cultural competency and cultural sensitivity principles. • Recognize the demographic, geographic, and ethnographic features within communities and populations when designing a clinical study. • Describe the relevance of cultural and population diversity in clinical research design. • Describe cultural and social variation in standards of research integrity. • Critique studies for evidence of health disparities, such as disproportional health effects on select populations (e.g., gender, age, ethnicity, race).
XI. Translational teamwork	• Build an interdisciplinary/intradisciplinary/ multidisciplinary team that matches the objectives of the research problem. • Manage an interdisciplinary team of scientists. • Advocate for multiple points of view. • Clarify language differences across disciplines. • Demonstrate group decision-making techniques. • Manage conflict. • Manage a clinical and/or translational research study.
XII. Leadership	• Work as a leader of a multidisciplinary research team. • Manage a multidisciplinary team across its fiscal, personnel, regulatory-compliance, and problem-solving requirements. • Maintain skills as mentor and mentee. • Validate others as a mentor. • Foster innovation and creativity.

continued

TABLE 1 Continued

Core Thematic Areas	Competencies
XIII. Cross-disciplinary training	• Apply principles of adult learning and competency-based instruction to educational activities. • Provide clinical and translational science instruction to beginning scientists. • Incorporate adult learning principles and mentoring strategies into interactions with beginning scientists and scholars in order to engage them in clinical and translational research. • Develop strategies for overcoming the unique curricular challenges associated with merging scholars from diverse backgrounds.
XIV. Community engagement	• Examine the characteristics that bind people together as a community, including social ties, common perspectives or interests, and geography. • Appraise the role of community engagement as a strategy for identifying community health issues, translating health research to communities, and reducing health disparities. • Summarize the principles and practices of the spectrum of community-engaged research. • Analyze the ethical complexities of conducting community-engaged research. • Specify how cultural and linguistic competence and health literacy have an impact on the conduct of community-engaged research.

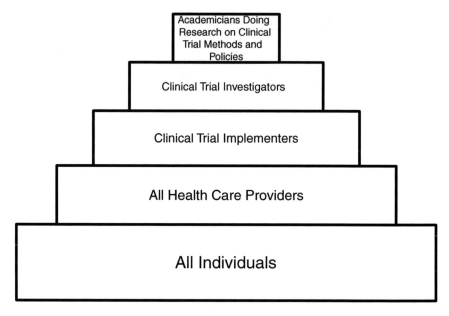

FIGURE 1 Workforce for a transformed clinical trials enterprise.

Appendix F

Discussion Paper[1]

Transforming the Economics of Clinical Trials

Judith M. Kramer, Duke University Medical Center, Clinical Trials Transformation Initiative, Duke Translational Medicine Institute; and Kevin A. Schulman, Duke University Medical Center, Fuqua School of Business, Duke Clinical Research Institute[2]

INTRODUCTION

Clinical trials are a means of gathering information about medical products or services. In medicine, however, they are also the fundamental means for advancing the underlying science and have enabled the many advances we have made in health care over the last few years. In many ways, clinical trials are the core infrastructure of the practice of medicine.

For an activity so vital to the field, the clinical research process is in serious trouble, especially in the United States. The cost of clinical trials for manufacturers of pharmaceuticals, biologics, and medical devices, as well as for public health investigators, continues to escalate. In pharmaceuticals (where this trend has been best documented), the costs have increased 7.4 percent annually over inflation for the last 20 years (DiMasi et al., 2003). The rising cost of clinical research is multifactorial but has been attributed to increased protocol complexity; an increase in local, regional, national, and international regulations/guidance and lack of harmoniza-

---

[1] The views expressed in this discussion paper are those of the authors and not necessarily of the authors' organizations or of the Institute of Medicine. The paper is intended to help inform and stimulate discussion. It has not been subjected to the review procedures of the Institute of Medicine and is not a report of the Institute of Medicine or of the National Research Council.

[2] Participants in the activities of the IOM Forum on Drug Discovery, Development, and Translation. This discussion paper was presented in draft form at the Forum's November 2011 workshop, Envisioning a Transformed Clinical Trials Enterprise in the United States: Establishing an Agenda for 2020, and finalized by the authors following the workshop.

tion among these; excessively risk-averse interpretations of regulations; and increasing time (and financial) pressures on clinician-investigators (Bollyky et al., 2010). Meanwhile, the need to conduct research in this environment has fueled the creation over the last three decades of a large and relatively new industry—clinical research organizations (CROs). While CROs improve efficiency for sponsors, their business practices also contribute to the current cost structure of clinical research. Irrespective of the factors driving the cost increases, the implications are clear. The greater the cost of research, the fewer new medical products that come to market, the less we know about the products that do, and the fewer initiated investigations of public health–inspired research questions. While we advance the concept of the "learning health care system" (Institute of Medicine [IOM], 2007), the cost of clinical research moves us further from this goal every day.

The Business of Clinical Trials

At its core, clinical research is not the practice of medicine but the collection of information about this practice. This conceptualization may provide some insight into the cost problem facing clinical research and could lead us to potential approaches for moving the clinical research effort onto a different cost trajectory. In other words, by viewing clinical research as an information and knowledge activity, we can look outside of medicine to understand the economics of information-intensive businesses in the United States.

In the information technology world, for example, Gordon Moore—co-founder of Intel—famously predicted in 1965 that the number of chips on a "minimal cost" transistor would double every 2 years (Moore, 1965); this massive increase in performance of the microchip over time has led to the reciprocal effect of dramatically reducing the cost of computers since the first personal computer was introduced in 1981. We have seen similar economic gains over time in other information-intensive industries, such as telecommunications (see Figure 1 for an estimate of improved productivity effects of health information technology) (Hillestad et al., 2005). The trajectory of cost in these information industries is driven by changes in both the technology and the underlying business models supporting the industry. Understanding this process is critical to our understanding of ways in which we can address the underlying cost issues in clinical research.

In his classic book *The Innovator's Dilemma*, Clay Christensen describes how new technology is brought to market by new companies through new business models, leading to cost and quality improvements over time (Christensen, 1997). He describes how cost and quality improvements in the computer disk–drive industry were driven by this creative destruction process in the marketplace. In reconceptualizing clinical research as the development of information about the practice of medicine, we can begin to lay out a plan for the transformation of the economics of clinical research that could mirror the cost trajectories found in other information industries. There are two components of this model—the core technology for clinical research and the core business model for clinical research.

A decade ago, clinical research relied largely on paper-based technology, in which site investigators would record their data on special, multipart case report forms (CRFs). These forms were collected centrally, entered into a database, and analyzed. The business process around clinical research entailed efforts to support this system to ensure that the data collected were accurate and valid. The cost of this model was related to the tremendous amount of labor involved in this exercise. Other costs were related to patient screening and recruitment to the trials.

Globalization of clinical research has evolved in part in response to the high unit costs of clinical research in developed economies, but it has not enabled the development of a different business model for clinical research (Glickman et al., 2009). Over the last decade, electronic data capture (EDC) has made some progress in transforming this model. In an EDC-enabled environment, paper forms are replaced by electronic forms, whereby sites enter their data into an electronic database. This technology has produced some efficiency gains as edit-checks reduce the cost of the manual data-query process. However, the EDC platform was largely embedded in the traditional clinical research business model, with legacy concepts around site monitoring and validation. New opportunities for central statistical monitoring of data in these systems were not widely embraced (Morrison et al., 2011). Patient screening and recruitment costs remained largely unchanged.

Over the next few years, providers will adopt electronic health records (EHRs) as a means of capturing data that are also critical to the clinical research process. Informatics can provide data-capture tools to create structured data forms in the medical records for research protocols, as well as data tools to allow aggregation of data across research sites. Because we can search clinical data repositories electronically to find eligible patients for research, for the first time EHR-enabled clinical research has the potential to reduce site-screening and recruitment costs of clinical research. The business framework for this type of clinical research enterprise has yet to be established.

A concurrent or subsequent research technology will be mobile-based technology that will allow direct contact with research subjects and direct data collection from patients. This technology could be paired with traditional clinical research processes or could enable a new model of direct-to-patient research efforts. The economics of this latter model of clinical research could be an order of magnitude less than current research costs.

Viewed in the timeframe of technology-enabled business models, we can make some general statements about the development of clinical research as an industry. While the technology for gathering clinical data for research has evolved over time, the business model supporting this technology clearly has not evolved with each stage of technology transformation. As a result, the potential economic opportunities from technology have been absorbed by legacy costs and processes shaped by previous generations of the business model for clinical research. These legacy costs exist in the sponsor organizations, in the regulatory environment, in the provider environment, and in the clinical research organizations themselves. In this context, innovation in technology has not generated the potential economic benefits that follow from business transformation. Further, hidden in this structure is the tremendous cost to sponsors of non–value-added processes within the clinical research environment that add tremendously to the cost of clinical research (Dilts and Sandler, 2006; DiMasi et al., 2003). The tremendous opportunity cost generated by lost productivity gains that would have been enabled by technology and business transformation over this time period is illustrated in Figure 2.

TRANSFORMING THE ECONOMICS OF CLINICAL TRIALS

This framework provides some insight into potential paths forward for the clinical research community. It implies an agenda of enabling business transformation with each generation of technology, requiring the retirement of outmoded business processes, and models to achieve economic transformation of clinical research. While this is a natural process in unregulated environments, this effort would need to take the form of a dedicated discipline in a regulated environment (Curtis and Schulman, 2006)·

As we consider approaches to enable business transformation that will keep pace with new technology and the escalating need for information about the practice of medicine, it would be wise to first articulate a common goal for the clinical research enterprise: to facilitate the efficient conduct of high-quality clinical trials to address pressing medical questions and evaluate therapeutic interventions. This goal serves both public health and business interests. In short, we want to do more trials at lower cost, complete them faster, and enhance their quality.

Engaging all sectors affected by clinical research in the conceptualization of new business models should facilitate the adoption of those new models. Although all sectors would likely support the overarching goal stated above, local concerns and incentives within individual sectors may prioritize maintenance of certain aspects of the existing business model over transformation of the research model. For the pharmaceutical, biological, and device industries, one might ask, "Why would a pharmaceutical company persist in conducting and funding clinical research activities that add cost but not value as measured by increased patient safety or reliability of data?" Understanding the lens through which actors assess the opportunity for business transformation will be critical to the success of this effort. Some suggest that, within the pharmaceutical industry, maintenance of activities that do not add value is not due to misinformation about the value of the activity but rather to avoidance of perceived regulatory risk—e.g., concern that a regulatory audit at a clinical site might delay or prevent approval of a product under development (which has a much greater cost to the sponsor) (Bollyky et al., 2010).

As technology evolves and industry sponsors, academicians, or the regulators themselves identify practices and guidelines based on outmoded business processes, collaborative initiatives such as the Sensible Guidelines group (Yusuf et al., 2008), the IOM Forum on Drug Discovery, Development, and Translation,[3] and the Clinical Trials Transformation Initiative (CTTI)[4] can engage regulators, industry, government researchers, academicians, and patients in conceptualizing and facilitating new business models. Active engagement to identify and overcome these issues will be critical in the regulated clinical research environment. Regulators can also help by clarifying any misperceptions of the current regulatory position, thereby providing reassurance to those afraid of migrating from the existing business model. Given the risks of business transformation for industry, these clarifications need to be as formal and timely as possible.

A recent example of such an approach to clinical trial monitoring is encouraging and may provide a prototype for a collaborative solution in the regulated environment. The cost of site management (monitoring) of clinical trials has been estimated to represent 25 to 30 percent of the cost of a clinical trial (Eisenstein et al., 2005). In a recent survey of 65 organizations that conduct or sponsor clinical trials, over 80 percent of responding pharmaceutical, biological, and device companies indicated that they always perform on-site monitoring visits and always perform source-document verification at the site. Despite over 80 percent of those companies reporting access to centrally available data to evaluate site performance, less than a quarter of them always used a centralized monitoring process to guide, target, or supplement site visits (Morrison et al., 2011).

---

[3] For more information on the work of the IOM Forum on Drug Discovery, Development, and Translation, visit http://www.iom.edu/Activities/Research/DrugForum.aspx.

[4] For more information on the projects of the Clinical Trials Transformation Initiative, visit https://www.ctti-clinicaltrials.org.

Despite a widespread perception that it is the regulators who require 100 percent source-document verification of all data items to ensure quality, a recent reflection paper from the European Medicines Agency (EMA) on risk-based quality management in clinical trials (EMA, 2011) and Food and Drug Administration (FDA) guidance for industry on a risk-based approach to monitoring (FDA, 2011) both clearly state otherwise. These regulatory documents acknowledged findings of the Sensible Guidelines group, CTTI, and other collaborative initiatives that influenced their recommendation of a risk-based solution to trial oversight. Both the EMA paper and the FDA's guidance embrace the use of centralized monitoring through real-time advanced data systems, consistent with the advantages of new technology.

The recent announcement by Pfizer of a clinical trial of a marketed product that will be conducted completely over the Internet (i.e., without identified clinical sites) was remarkable for the fact that the sponsor and the FDA worked very closely with the principal investigator to design and test this new approach for reliability and safety (Mansell, 2011). This model suggests an alternative pathway that can provide a more timely response to sponsors to address questions about new research business models.

It would be worthwhile also to consider the local cultural and financial incentives of academic and government institutions that engage in clinical research and clinical care. If clinical research is the collection of information about the practice of medicine, new technology and business models that promote efficiency should enable many more clinical questions to be addressed and enable more potential savings by identifying expensive but ineffective interventions. It is striking that the health care system has developed so that its business model can conflict financially with improvements in the practice of medicine. For example, many institutions pursued aggressive programs for high-dose chemotherapy and stem-cell transplantation for breast cancer before the definitive clinical evidence was developed indicating lack of efficacy of this treatment for breast cancer (Schulman et al., 2003). Leadership at the institutional level must ensure that the financial interests of the local institution do not overpower the public health interest in generating evidence to drive the practice of medicine.

There is also an issue of "sunk costs" from the perspective of an institution, or decision making guided by past investment strategies in clinical research. For instance, once an academic institution has invested in creating a smoothly functioning institutional review board (IRB) and an electronic system for protocol submissions to the IRB, officials at that institution may be reluctant to defer to central IRBs for industry-sponsored multicenter trials being conducted at their institution due to concern about the loss of financial support for their own infrastructure. While these concerns are valid, business transformation requires the discipline to jettison these investments when better opportunities arise. Obviously, this discipline for creative destruction of old models is not a core competency within the health care system. New business models may be thwarted if these concerns are not directly addressed.

An overall approach to ensure that the business model keeps pace with new technology and information needs should start with an agenda for research on how we do research. This agenda should be dedicated to addressing the potential issues in business transformation with each stage of technology migration. This effort requires a clear statement of the goals of different steps in the research process and an understanding of the regulatory and business processes that support each of these steps. The research agenda will then review the potential transformation of these steps given the next generation of technology. This could include recasting goals, transforming regulations, and transforming business processes. The goals of this agenda should be forward-looking rather than focused on refining the current environment. This agenda should be driven by a goal of transforming the clinical research environment every 2 to 5 years, which will lead to tremendous improvements in the economic efficiency of clinical research.

While the research will highlight pathways to business-process transformation, implementing this collaborative approach to business-process improvement is antithetical to the usual business transformation. Incumbent business models inherently fight business-process transformation when given the opportunity, either consciously or unconsciously. Experience is used to argue for the current business model with regulators, and, in the absence of organizations representing business transformation, this acts as a potent force. The concept of a forward-looking research agenda is one means of mitigating this natural response of incumbent organizations. Dedicating part of the regulatory structure to support this agenda would be another means of advancing this goal (i.e., safe harbors for business-process innovation could be a critical enabling strategy). Organizing the clinical community to enable these changes would also be a critical step in this process (e.g., business transformation could include removing clinicians or nurses from some of their current roles in the research process).

Although clinical research clearly provides information that underpins the practice of medicine, more education about clinical research is needed for health professionals. A recent report on the ClinicalTrials.gov results database raised concerns about the quality of some submitted entries, which may relate directly to insufficient knowledge on the part of investigators about fundamental precepts of clinical research—e.g., 20 percent of trials with recorded results reported more than two primary outcome measures, and 5 percent of trials reported more than five primary outcome measures (Zarin et al., 2011). Education about clinical research is necessary to ensure the ability to develop well-designed clinical research protocols, to maximize practitioners' and patients' participation in trials, to produce clinicians capable of competently interpreting and applying the results of completed trials, and to help facilitate new models of clinical research. These skills should become part of essential knowledge of the clinical care community and the core of the learning health care system. Health care professionals trained in clinical research can more competently analyze and streamline complex regulatory and administrative processes for clinical research within institutions to facilitate the adoption of new business models.

CONCLUSION

The economic crisis in clinical research is driven by the inability to transform the business model for research as the core informatics technology evolves. A concerted, multi-stakeholder effort to address adoption of new business models for clinical research is a critical step in unlocking the potential economic transformation of clinical research in the coming decade.

REFERENCES

Bollyky, T. J., I. M. Cockburn, and E. Berndt. 2010. Bridging the gap: Improving clinical development and the regulatory pathways for health products for neglected diseases. *Clinical Trials* 7:719-734.

Christensen, C. M. 1997. *The Innovator's Dilemma*. Cambridge, MA: Harvard Business Press.

Curtis, L. H., and K. A. Schulman. 2006. Overregulation of health care: Musings on disruptive innovation theory. *Law and Contemporary Problems* 69:195-206.

Dilts, D. M., and A. B. Sandler. 2006. Invisible barriers to clinical trials: The impact of structural, infrastructural, and procedural barriers to opening oncology clinical trials. *Journal of Clinical Oncology* 24:4545-4552.

DiMasi, J.A., R. W. Hansen, and H. G. Grabowski. 2003. The price of innovation: New estimates of drug development costs. *Journal of Health Economics* 22:151-185.

Eisenstein, E. L., P. W. Lemons II, B. E. Tardiff, K. A. Schulman, M. K. Jolly, and R. M. Califf. 2005. Reducing the costs of phase III cardiovascular clinical trials. *American Heart Journal* 149:482-488.

EMA (European Medicines Agency). 2011. *Reflection Paper on Risk Based Quality Management in Clinical Trials*. http://www.ema.europa.eu/docs/en_GB/document_library/Scientific_guideline/2011/08/WC500110059.pdf (accessed October 2, 2011).

FDA (Food and Drug Administration). 2011. *Guidance for Industry Oversight of Clinical Investigations—A Risk-Based Approach to Monitoring* [Draft]. http://www.fda.gov/downloads/Drugs/GuidanceComplianceRegulatoryInformation/Guidances/UCM269919.pdf (accessed October 2, 2011).

Glickman, S. W., J. G. McHutchison, E. D. Peterson, C. B. Cairns, R. A. Harrington, R. M. Califf, and K. A. Schulman. 2009. Ethical and scientific implications of the globalization of clinical research. *New England Journal of Medicine* 360:816-823.

Hillestad, R., J. Bigelow, A. Bower, F. Girosi, R. Meili, R. Scoville, and R. Taylor. 2005. Can electronic medical record system transform health care? Potential health benefits, savings, and costs. *Health Affairs* 24:1103-1117.

IOM (Institute of Medicine). 2007. *The Learning Healthcare System: Workshop Summary.* Washington, DC: The National Academies Press.

Mansell, P. 2011. Pfizer announces "virtual" clinical trial pilot in US. *Pharma Times Online,* June 9. http://www.pharmatimes.com/article/11-06-09/Pfizer_announces_virtual_clinical_trial_pilot_in_US.aspx. (accessed September 12, 2011).

Moore, G. 1965. Cramming more components onto integrated circuits. *Electronics Magazine,* April 19.

Morrison, B. W., C. J. Cochran, J. G. White, J. Harley, C. F. Kleppinger, A. Liu, J. T. Mitchel, D. F. Nickerson, C. R. Zacharias, J. M. Kramer, and J. D. Neaton. 2011. Monitoring the quality of conduct of clinical trials: A survey of current practices. *Clinical Trials* 8:342-349.

Schulman, K. A., E. A. Stadtmauer, S. D. Reed, H. A. Glick, L. J. Goldstein, J. M. Pines, J. A. Jackman, S. Suzuki, M. J. Styler, P. A. Crilley, T. R. Klumpp, K. F. Mangan, and J. H. Glick. 2003. Economic analysis of conventional-dose chemotherapy compared with high-dose chemotherapy plus autologous hematopoietic stem-cell transplantation for metastatic breast cancer. *Bone Marrow Transplant* 31:205-210.

Yusuf, S., J. Bosch, P. J. Devereaux, R. Collins, C. Baigent, C. Granger, R. Califf, and R. Temple. 2008. Sensible guidelines for the conduct of large randomized trials. *Clinical Trials* 5:38-39.

Zarin, D. A., T. Tse, R. J. Williams, R. M. Califf, and N. C. Ide. 2011. The ClinicalTrials.gov results database: Update and key issues. *New England Journal of Medicine* 364:852-860.

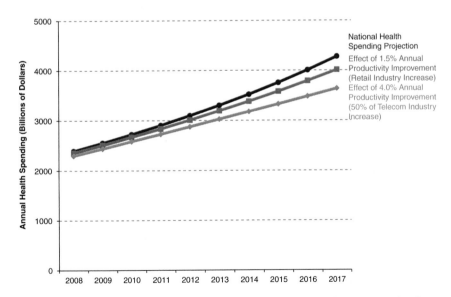

FIGURE 1 Possible improved productivity effects of health information technology. SOURCE: Adapted from Hillestad et al., 2005.

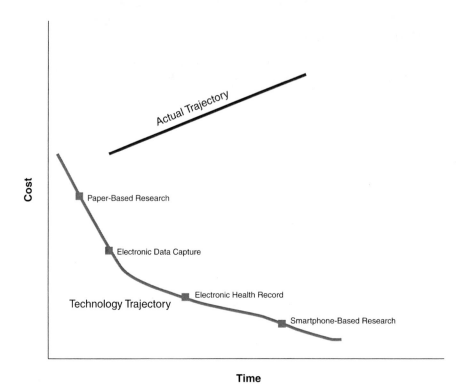

FIGURE 2 Cost trajectory in clinical trials. Figure depicts the opportunity cost (area between the two curves) generated from lost productivity gains that would have been enabled by technology and business transformation over time.
SOURCE: Kevin Schulman and Preethi Sama, Duke University.

Appendix G

Discussion Paper[1]

Developing a Clinical Trials Infrastructure

Paul Eisenberg, Amgen, Inc.; Petra Kaufmann, National Institute of Neurological Disorders and Stroke; Ellen Sigal, Friends of Cancer Research; and Janet Woodcock, U.S. Food and Drug Administration[2]

INTRODUCTION

Clinical trials in the United States have a rich history of involving academic, industry, and government institutions (e.g. the National Institutes of Health [NIH]) to address important medical questions. Nonetheless, over time, clinical trials in the United States have become too expensive, difficult to enroll, inefficient to implement, and ineffective to support the development of new medical products using modern evidentiary standards. The nation's capacity for conducting clinical trials is also inadequate to provide the evidence needed for rational clinical practice. For instance, clinical practice guidelines are routinely issued by professional societies but only a small proportion of these guidelines are based on high-quality evidence from randomized trials (Lee and Vielemeyer, 2011; Tricoci et al., 2009). Furthermore, there is a growing recognition that patients and other stakeholders need to be partners in the development, conduct, and interpretation of clinical trials. Importantly, commu-

[1] The views expressed in this discussion paper are those of the authors and not necessarily of the authors' organizations or of the Institute of Medicine. The paper is intended to help inform and stimulate discussion. It has not been subjected to the review procedures of the Institute of Medicine and is not a report of the Institute of Medicine or of the National Research Council.

[2] Participants in the activities of the IOM Forum on Drug Discovery, Development, and Translation. This discussion paper was presented in draft form at the Forum's November 2011 workshop, Envisioning a Transformed Clinical Trials Enterprise in the United States: Establishing an Agenda for 2020, and finalized by the authors following the workshop.

nity medical practitioners and other important caregivers (for example, clinical psychologists) provide an avenue for partnering with patients but largely do not participate in clinical trials as investigators or as practitioners willing to refer their patients to trials. This diminishes patient access to trials and decreases the generalizability or "real-world" relevance of trials that are conducted.

Clinical trials have been funded and sponsored by NIH, other government agencies, academic groups, voluntary health organizations, and industry. The infrastructure to support the trials is often developed specifically for a given trial or in a sponsor-specific manner, with the exception of trials performed by cooperative groups or other organized structures, including NIH's AIDS Clinical Trials Group [ACTG] network at the National Institute of Allergy and Infectious Diseases and the Cancer Therapy Evaluation Program [CTEP] at the National Cancer Institute, as well as networks set up by patient groups (e.g., the Cystic Fibrosis Foundation and others). Investigators and staff may be recruited for the purposes of a specific trial only, and the team is disbanded after trial completion. Efforts to develop a consistent infrastructure for clinical trials have been limited in scope, often considering only issues of investigator or patient recruitment. Although there are examples of more expansive approaches to developing an infrastructure (e.g., adverse event reporting conventions in cancer studies), in general these efforts have not translated into harmonized national or international efforts. As a result, there are few clinical research structures in the United States that combine mature clinical trials infrastructure, experienced staff, and established procedures that also have access to large numbers of patients with a specific disease or disorder.

Over the past decade, factors including the increased number and size of clinical trials to support the development of pharmaceutical agents have resulted in a shift to international multicenter trials in which patients are recruited through open enrollment as a global effort. Since the United States constitutes only 5 percent of the world's population and provides one of the most expensive and least efficient clinical trials enterprises, it is not surprising that many trials have a very small representation of U.S. participants, or none at all. This has raised concern with respect to the applicability of the results to patients in the United States and whether the human-subject protections and overall quality of international multicenter trials is equivalent to trials that are performed in the United States.

Development of an explicit and transparent national clinical trials infrastructure may potentially increase access to clinical trials for multiple stakeholders. For example, training and recruitment of less-experienced investigators who practice in settings that are relevant to the clinical questions being addressed may improve the applicability of the results to the issues being studied. In addition to improving the ultimate applicability and uptake of clinical trial results, these community-based investigators could provide important expertise, in partnership with patients, in developing innovative clinical trial designs that efficiently study outcomes that are of interest to patients and the public. Patient access to clinical trials may also be improved by taking advantage of nontraditional means for awareness and enrollment, such as web-based trials and the use of social media.

An appropriately implemented infrastructure for clinical trials would recognize the value of participation in trials in the continuous improvement of health care. Quality improvement and evidence-based medicine require the discipline of clinical investigation as an integral component of successful implementation. A key objective of health care reform in the United States is to encourage use of the most effective therapies and implementation strategies. This will require multiple types of clinical trials conducted in many different settings. Academic centers that are involved in clinical trials often take advantage of the infrastructure that is created to address clinical questions. In contrast, nonacademic practitioners and institutions may not have the processes and support to use clinical trial methodology in quality improvement. Broader access to clinical trial expertise may be necessary to conduct trials in real-world settings, evaluate special populations, and understand the long-term consequences of interventions.

Development of a clinical trials infrastructure can only be a component of the solution to the issues highlighted, but the potential of key initiatives to support or catalyze change in the clinical trials capacity and quality in the United States is worth considering and is the topic of this discussion paper. It is also worth considering that while electronic health records, standard nomenclature, and data standards clearly are critical to an efficient and scalable infrastructure, these efforts remain immature with respect to broad implementation in the U.S. health care system. Accordingly, the following discussion topics are proposed:

- What would constitute an optimal clinical trials infrastructure in the United States?
- How would such an infrastructure address the problems stated above? Should infrastructure solutions be universal, tailored to specific research settings, or integrated through common standards?
- What would be required to develop a clinical trials infrastructure? What is achievable in the near- versus long-term?

ELEMENTS OF AN OPTIMAL CLINICAL TRIALS INFRASTRUCTURE IN THE UNITED STATES

Although the sponsor, investigators, and purpose of clinical trials vary considerably, there are common underlying components that can be considered with respect to potential for a clinical trials infrastructure in the United States to enhance quality and reduce the cost of clinical trials. Specifically, the following key common elements are required for most clinical trials, with the exception of non-interventional studies where certain components listed below are not necessary. These components could provide the framework for a sustainable and continuous clinical trials infrastructure:

- Investigator recruitment
- Experienced clinical trial personnel
- Protocol development support
- Regulatory approval to conduct the clinical trial (e.g., Investigational New Drug [IND] applications in the United States)
- Good Clinical Practice (GCP) requirements (primarily for interventional clinical trials), including
  — informed consent,
  — ethical review,
  — human research participant protections,
  — privacy considerations,
  — investigator training and qualifications, and
  — adverse event (AE) reporting
- Contractual agreements between sponsors, institutions, and investigators
- Participant recruitment plan
- Coordination of clinical trial investigators and centers both in the United States and globally
- Quality-control systems to ensure GCP compliance
- Data collection, management, and analysis
- Data standards (e.g., medical concept coding, diagnosis coding, data standards)
- Communication of results (publication)
- Registration of clinical trials and results on ClinicalTrials.gov

POTENTIAL AREAS THAT A NATIONAL CLINICAL TRIALS INFRASTRUCTURE COULD ADDRESS

Investigator Training

- *Standardized core content and the availability of Continuing Medical Education (CME) credits for clinical investigator training.* Standardized online training and certification would avoid the redundancy of many trial performance sites each developing their own training programs. Also, investigators participating in multiple initiatives could satisfy the training requirements periodically for all projects they are working on and physician-investigators could receive CME credit for their participation in clinical research.

- *Centralized certification processes for clinical investigators.* A central online training and certification system as described above would allow sponsors and institutions to centrally verify that participating investigators meet the training and expertise requirements of a given project.

Investigator Recruitment

- *Information technology (IT) solutions for matching investigators to sponsors.* If central online information could be available on the expertise, capacity, resources, and patient access of potential trial sites, this would be a good initial step in assisting with site selection. The number of patients with a given condition who are potential trial participants is typically overestimated. To address this, these data could be drawn in a de-identified manner from clinical databases such as electronic medical records (EMRs) or billing records.

- *Development of investigator networks, primary care versus specialty/ academic care.* The relationship of the infrastructure with respect to investigator recruitment, training, and support will be important in the development of clinical research networks. For example, investigators in the primary care setting typically are identified by geographical proximity to academic centers. The infrastructure to support investigators in this circumstance would likely be coordinated by the core center. However, a web-based strategy for developing an investigator network is less dependent on geographical concerns or central academic support and would allow investigators to self-organize. However, in both methods for identifying investigators, common approaches to training and certification would facilitate the development of the network.

- *Development of novel approaches to clinical trial development.* For example, clinical questions or concepts could be placed in an online site where potential investigators or sponsors could propose potential trials. This model would allow patients and other stakeholders to propose questions to be answered through clinical trials. Engaging patients in the identification of key research questions that are important to them could also help facilitate their participation and enrollment in clinical trials (Institute of Medicine [IOM], 2012). NIH, industry, academia, professional societies, voluntary health associations, and patient advocacy groups could facilitate this partnership between patients and researchers. An online trial infrastructure would serve many stakeholders. Therefore, this could be done in partnership among private and potentially government organizations.

Investigator/Clinical Trial Staff Support

Lack of coordinators/administrative support is one of the barriers to engaging physicians outside of academic centers to participate as investigators in clinical trials. Expansion of the investigator network for clinical trials should consider approaches to supporting these activities. A flexible infrastructure to provide clinical research coordination and administrative support for clinical trials should be considered along with many of the similar training and certification elements for investigators. Some of the areas in which support is needed for the various components of a clinical trial include the following:

- *Standardized contracts* are key to accelerating the contracting and subcontracting in clinical trials, as contracting typically causes the greatest delays in start-up. Posting trial agreements transparently online and pre-negotiating master trial agreements between potential sponsors and networks can accelerate the start-up of trials as only the few project-specific issues would then have to be negotiated.

- *Standardized approach to reimbursable medical expenses.* It would be helpful if a standard fee schedule for clinical research tasks was available, adjusted for regional and local differences in cost, for example, adjusted in relationship to Medicare or Medicaid payments.

- *Management of privacy issues to facilitate observational trials.*

Regulatory Approval

- Development of *a globally harmonized regulatory database, nomenclature, and identification of clinical trials* involving investigational molecules or devices and encouraging regulatory authorities to use this database in facilitating regulatory approval.

- *Centralized institutional review board (IRB) review* for multicenter projects enhances human subjects' protection. The often serial and circular review of one protocol at multiple sites typically does not add value to the ethics review. Multicenter trials should designate an IRB of record to provide a review. After passing the initial review at the central IRB, the near-final protocol should be sent to the participating institutions for comments within 2 weeks. These comments should be provided by a designated institutional official, but not a full IRB. This allows for the exceptional modification of the consent or protocol to adjust to local context, but will avoid the delays that arise from multiple IRB reviews.

Recruiting Clinical Trial Participants

- *Patient education* is very important to successful trial recruitment. This includes education of the general public as to the need for clinical trials to bring better treatments to people. There are already several online and print resources on clinical trials in general.

- *Disease-specific and consumer friendly solutions for aggregating clinical trial reporting may improve the understanding of the value of participating in clinical trials.* As an example, an individual or health care professional could opt-in to get disease-specific clinical trial information that aggregates ClinicalTrials.gov data and literature reports and provides links to trials and investigators that are recruiting patients. The service could be paid for by the trial sponsors that are recruiting. However, regulatory implications for sponsors and the assurance that accurate information is provided to the public would need to be addressed.

- *Pre-identification of individuals interested in clinical trials.* If people could indicate their interest in trial participation, trial recruitment could be facilitated. Ways to indicate an interest could include carrying a document similar to an advanced directive or patients being asked at hospital admission or at check-in at an outpatient office if they would like information on trial opportunities. It could also include carrying a card, similar to an organ donor card, identifying an interest in participating in research.

- *Integration of electronic health records with clinical trial databases* would be another means of improving clinical trial recruitment and also developing realistic estimates of potential patients available for specific trials. Patients could be offered an opt-in approach to be made aware of clinical trials for which they might be eligible as part of a health care system interaction. Physicians could also be provided with alerts when patients meet criteria for enrollment in a clinical trial. Examples of the latter have been successfully implemented by some investigators based on laboratory data or other electronic medical information.

- *Developing a patient-friendly interface with ClinicalTrials.gov.* Online information on the availability of trials would be helpful so that patients, their families, and their physicians could more easily find information on trial opportunities. ClinicalTrials.gov is an excellent and complete resource of trial information. However, it was not designed to help find trial opportunities. If a patient-friendly "front porch" to ClinicalTrials.gov could be created that would use the high-quality and up-to-date information on ClinicalTrials.gov but make it searchable—for example, by disease, geographic location, and basic entry criteria for the trial—this could become a very useful tool for patient education and clinical trial recruitment efforts. Other approaches could include use of social media or "opt-in" for clinical trial information triggered by health care or pharmacy interactions. Transparent communication of clinical trials results should be automated and reliable in order to increase visibility into the clinical trials enterprise. ClinicalTrials.gov has increased transparency in the clinical trials enterprise with regard to the registration of trials along with their key characteristics (including population, sample size, entry criteria, and primary outcomes). More recently, the reporting of results has been added to the registry. These results are transparently communicated, but provided at a level that is not aimed at patients and the public. A lay abstract describing the results could be provided through a "patient portal." An IT system to provide specific information on trial opportunities could be created in partnership with industry, the public sector, and patient groups.

Conducting Clinical Trials

- *Clinical trial identifier standards for identification of patients/trials in EMRs.* EMRs should include codes for clinical research. When possible, harmonized data standards for use in clinical research should be mapped to electronic health records to facilitate screening.

- Development of a *centralized electronic tool for notifying investigators, regulators, and IRBs* of AEs, "Dear Investigator" letters, and clinical trial amendments.

- *Online protocol-authoring tools and templates* can help create more uniform protocol formats and thus facilitate the correct implementation of research protocols by research staff who are often involved in several protocols at a given site. Online protocol systems can also facilitate the central management of amendments and communication.

- *Global harmonization of regulatory requirements for AE reporting to agencies, investigators, and IRBs to reduce clinical trial complexity and cost.* Adoption of the Development Safety Update Report will also facilitate a uniform approach to assessment and reporting of safety issues.

- *Continued development of guidance documents relating to clinical trial design, endpoints, and other key considerations is critical.* In addition, revision of guidance documents to update recommendations should be done in a timely fashion and include external stakeholder input. Cross-stakeholder forums should be developed to review clinical trial metrics (e.g., the utility of various clinical trial designs) with a focus on improving the efficiency of the clinical trials enterprise.

- *Advance fit-for-purpose AE reporting.* Alignment of global AE reporting to regulators vs. investigators could increase the efficiency and effectiveness of clinical trials, especially trials conducted at multiple international sites. The burden of AE reporting to investigators and IRBs could be reduced by focusing on significant new safety information and periodic aggregate summary reports.

- *Online management of informed consent and informed consent updates.* Similarly, informed consent templates could be managed and shared online. Overall, consent forms would benefit from simpler, shorter language.

WHAT WOULD BE REQUIRED?

One model for a clinical trials infrastructure involves organizing disease-specific networks that include medical practitioners in the community. These networks would not be designed to evaluate a single agent, but rather to evaluate a series of interventions, including investigational therapies or preventives. Standardized data collection and protocols to reduce costs would be essential. Inclusion of community practitioners with the appropriate support and this infrastructure could increase patient access to trials, trial accrual, and engagement of the medical community in evidence-based medicine. Increasingly, practitioners are aligned with local or regional health care systems—both public and privately run. Ideally, such systems would participate in and support clinical trials on problems important to their community as part of quality improvement.

When the creation of disease-specific networks does not make sense because of the resource requirements—which may be challenging in the current environment for less common diseases or for indications in which few trials take place—other alternatives may be more feasible. For example, the Clinical and Translational Science Awards (CTSA) consortium of 60 medical research institutions across the nation could organize clinical trial networks across a broad range of diseases. Alternatively, these networks could focus on a group of diseases or a particular population (e.g., children). In all cases, community practitioners should be supported to participate by provision of training and logistical and administrative support. A "virtual coordinator" could remotely support several community practice sites in a clinical trial network. Another approach is a "hub and spoke" system in which a larger medical center would partner with community health care providers on designing and implementing clinical trials.

How could such networks be supported? Funding such an enterprise in the face of current budgetary constraints is the primary issue. Ongoing costs could be mitigated by the use of consortia, contribution of disease groups, and fee-for-service arrangements for evaluation of new technologies. However, existing structures, including CTSAs, health care systems, and academic medicine, do not have sufficient resources to dedicate to creation of a trials network, nor is this seen as part of their core mission. Despite these problems, the question remains: how can the United States afford not to have a clinical trials infrastructure? As the cost of health care continues to rise, advances in basic biomedical science envision new interventions, and the costs of medical product development soar, an effective, efficient, and reliable mechanism for generating evidence on the value of health care must be seen as a necessity, not an option. We cannot afford to continue without the means to generate a solid evidence base for medical practice.

REFERENCES

Institute of Medicine (IOM). 2012. *Public Engagement and Clinical Trials: New Models and Disruptive Technologies: Workshop Summary.* Washington, DC: The National Academies Press.

Lee, D. H., and O. Vielemeyer. 2011. Analysis of overall level of evidence behind Infectious Diseases Society of America practice guidelines. *Ann Intern Med* 171:18-22.

Tricoci P., J. M. Allen, J. M. Kramer, R. M. Califf, and S. C. Smith Jr. 2009. Scientific evidence underlying the ACC/AHA clinical practice guidelines. *JAMA* 301:831-841.

Appendix H

Discussion Paper[1]

Canadian Strategy on Patient-Oriented Research

Jean L. Rouleau, Institute of Circulatory and Respiratory Health,
Canadian Institutes of Health and Research; Penny Moody-Corbett,
Strategy on Patient-Oriented Research,
Canadian Institutes of Health and Research[2]

In Canada, as elsewhere, the translation of health research outcomes to development of products and services for health care and final implementation in patients does not progress as rapidly, efficiently, or successfully as it should. In order to address this problem, Canada has embarked on a bold new strategy to improve health care and health care delivery based on evidence from research outcomes and integration of knowledge to the policy makers and users. The Strategy on Patient-Oriented Research (SPOR) is a pan-Canadian program involving health researchers and professionals, policy makers, and patients. It is a partnership led by a national steering committee which is co-chaired by the president of the Canadian Institutes of Health Research, the leading funder of health research in Canada, and the president and chief scientific officer of the University Health Network, one of Canada's leading hospitals and research institutes, and includes membership from all levels of government, the private

---

[1] The views expressed in this discussion paper are those of the authors and not necessarily of the authors' organizations or of the Institute of Medicine. The paper is intended to help inform and stimulate discussion. It has not been subjected to the review procedures of the Institute of Medicine and is not a report of the Institute of Medicine or of the National Research Council.

[2] Participants in the activities of the IOM Forum on Drug Discovery, Development, and Translation. This discussion paper is based on a submission to the Forum's November 2011 workshop, Envisioning a Transformed Clinical Trials Enterprise in the United States: Establishing an Agenda for 2020, to inform the workshop discussions surrounding international case studies in the area of clinical research transformation.

sector, health charities, health science networks, universities, and patient advocacy. The goal of the Canadian patient-oriented research strategy is to improve health outcomes and enhance patient's health care experience based on translation of research outcomes into the health care system.

The Strategy consists of four major objectives:

1. Improvement of the human health research environment and infrastructure.
2. Establishment of mechanisms to better train and mentor health professionals and non-clinicians in health research.
3. Improvement of organizational, regulatory, and financial support for multisite studies.
4. Integration of best practices into the health care system.

In order to improve the human research environment and infrastructure in Canada, SPOR will help develop specialized Patient-Oriented Research Networks (hereafter, Networks) and specialized research service centers referred to as Support for People and Patient-Oriented Research and Trials (SUPPORT) units. The Networks will be led by a team of principal investigators with internationally recognized research credentials and health systems/delivery expertise. The Networks will be national in scope and will bring together a unified group to build a critical mass of technical and scientific expertise to provide research leadership in an effort to improve the delivery of care through the development and validation of health care interventions. The Networks will be focused in specialty areas of national importance (e.g., mental health, community-based primary health care, etc.) as judged by the national steering committee, and the Networks will work with international partners to generate evidence on best practices for patient care in the community. Through mentoring and training, the Networks will provide the tools for the next generation of health researchers to better integrate research with improved health care and health care delivery.

In order to ensure nationally distributed health research services and expertise, SUPPORT units will be developed and housed in each of the provinces or regions of the country. The SUPPORT units will provide the personnel and infrastructure to support large-scale multi-site national and international studies involving patients and/or patient records. The units will themselves be centres of research excellence and opportunity, provided through senior research chairs with specializations in areas such as health research methodologies, health systems research, and knowledge translation. The SUPPORT units will include people with expertise to design, analyze, and manage large-scale, multisite studies (e.g., biostatisticians, epidemiologists, health economists, etc.). The SUPPORT units will offer consultation services for the research community which will be provided by qualified personnel and trainees who will gain practical experience in this work environment while providing support to the research community. Expertise from the SUPPORT units will be available for local and regional health initiatives. Nationally, the SPOR initiative will ensure common approaches for SUPPORT units across the country and thereby enhance the ability of Canadian researchers to engage in large national studies, such as those initiated by the SPOR Networks (see Figure 1). It is anticipated that the SUPPORT units will be recognized internationally as an access point to the Canadian patient-centered research community.

Health researchers and policy developers recognize the advantages as well as the challenges of doing research in Canada. As in other international jurisdictions, it is acknowledged that complex organizational, regulatory, and financial support for clinical and health research can act as barriers to effective research or implementation of research outcomes. In order to address these areas, SPOR has established external advisory committees that will provide specific direction or guidance for improved or coordinated national activities. For example, over the past 6 months, Canada has embarked on a common contracts pilot program facilitated by the Canadian Institutes of Health Research, Rx&D (the umbrella organization for the Canadian pharmaceutical industry) and the Association of Canadian Academic Healthcare Organizations. External advisory committees have been established to address topics that will simplify and focus clinical research reporting and develop more flexible and adaptive protocols; streamline the process of research ethics review, in particular for multisite studies, and provide appropriate infrastructure and access for the rich source of population and administrative data and electronic records in Canada. In addition, an external advisory committee exists to develop a strategy for students and young scholars, both clinical and nonclinical, wishing to pursue careers in the field of patient-oriented research.

The success of initiatives like SPOR in resolving the multiple challenges facing patient-oriented research in Canada relies upon many factors, some of which are specific to Canada. SPOR has three characteristics that, although present in other national and international initiatives, have perhaps received greater attention in Canada's initiative. First, all programs require partnerships and buy-in from the community in order to assure alignment of all stakeholders and to optimize coherence and impact. Partners include federal and provincial governments, academic institutions such as academic health science networks, universities and institutes, life science industries, charities, funding agencies and, indeed, all health research–related stakeholders. Second, in order to optimize coherence and impact, the SPOR program is a comprehensive one that attempts to cluster the multiple challenges and solutions facing patient-oriented research under one umbrella. And third, SPOR proposes a major focus on developing clinical research efforts addressing the needs for improving the quality and efficiency of our health care system.

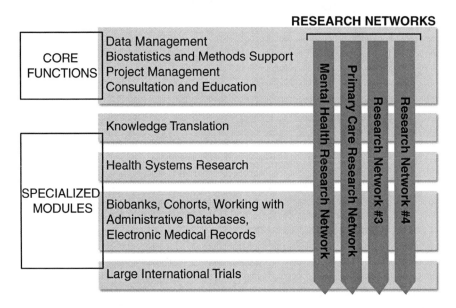

FIGURE 1 Relationship between SUPPORT units and Research Networks: When combined, SUPPORT units will provide the infrastructure and skills for highly specialized Research Networks to identify and tackle key clinical questions. The primary focus of Research Networks #3 and #4 has not yet been decided by the national steering committee.

Appendix I

Discussion Paper[1]

Health Research as a Public Good

Michael D. Rawlins, Academy of Medical Sciences Working Group on the Regulation and Governance of Health Research[2]

The arrangements for the regulation and governance of health research in the United Kingdom (UK) have evolved, piecemeal, over the past 30 years, and much is now enshrined in UK and European Union (EU) legislation. Each individual measure was introduced with the best of intentions, but the law of unintended consequences has meant that the regulatory and governance framework for health research is now dysfunctional, uncoordinated, and no longer "fit for purpose." The EU directive regulating clinical trials places unnecessary and unreasonable burdens on investigators; there are at least a dozen bodies involved in granting ethical approval for health research; and each National Health Service (NHS) hospital involved in a study insists on re-examining the ethical, legal, and financial arrangements that have already been largely scrutinised by one (and often more) of the relevant ethics committees.

---

[1] The views expressed in this discussion paper are those of the authors and not necessarily of the authors' organizations or of the Institute of Medicine. The paper is intended to help inform and stimulate discussion. It has not been subjected to the review procedures of the Institute of Medicine and is not a report of the Institute of Medicine or of the National Research Council.

[2] Participant in the activities of the IOM Forum on Drug Discovery, Development, and Translation. This discussion paper is based on a submission to the Forum's November 2011 workshop, Envisioning a Transformed Clinical Trials Enterprise in the United States: Establishing an Agenda for 2020, to inform the workshop discussions surrounding international case studies in the area of clinical research transformation.

BOX 1
Guiding Principles for the Regulation and
Governance of Health Research

1. Safeguard the well-being of research participants
2. Facilitate high-quality health research for public benefit
3. Be proportionate, efficient, and coordinated
4. Build and maintain confidence in the conduct and relevance of health research through transparency, clarity, accountability, and contestability

---

The goal of health research—encompassing experimental medicine, clinical trials, and epidemiology—is to improve and sustain the public's health. Whether involving healthy volunteers, patients, or the public more widely, the Academy of Medical Sciences (2011) has enunciated four fundamental principles (see Box 1) that should underpin the regulatory environment for health research.

In the United Kingdom, however, none of these principles is fully (and in many instances even partially) met. Even Principle 1—safeguarding the well-being of research participants—is undermined by the mindless controls that are too often imposed and that lead to a false sense of security. Principles 2, 3, and 4 are observed in the breach. Yet we know that the public, in the United Kingdom, has an appetite for research. Most patients, given the opportunity, want to take part in clinical trials. Half a million members of the general public have contributed their personal details (in anonymised form), as well as blood, urine, and saliva, to UK Biobank. In order to meet the aspirations of patients, the public, and the health research community (including both the life sciences industries and academic investigators), the following measures are being taken:

1. In response to the advice of the Academy of Medical Sciences' report, the government has created (as of December 1, 2011) a Health Research Agency (HRA). In line with the academy's proposals, it is intended that this new body fulfill two functions. First, it will bring together the current disparate arrangements for providing ethics approvals for health research. The National Research Ethics Service has already moved into the HRA and other bodies will do so shortly. Some of the arrangements for ethics review are enshrined in primary legislation and will take a little time to unravel, but there is a real determination, on the part of the government, to ensure that rapid progress is made. Second, the Academy of Medical Sciences expects the HRA to coordinate the research

governance arrangements in individual NHS hospitals. For multi-centre studies a "lead" institution could take responsibility for the global checks, leaving individual hospitals to confirm the availability of patients and staff time. Consortia of individual NHS hospitals have already started to do this. Alternatively or additionally, the HRA could itself undertake the global checks. Whatever arrangements that emerge, individual hospitals—as independent legal entities—will need to agree, formally, to take part in particular studies. It will therefore be incumbent on the new agency to earn and retain the confidence of the NHS hospitals themselves as well as the wider research community and the public.

2. In its report on the current climate for health research, the academy was highly critical of both the principles and the operational details of the EU's Clinical Trials Directive. This directive is overburdensome (including so-called "non-investigational" studies that have no place in the context of drug regulation), disproportionate, and applied inconsistently across the European Union. As a member state of the European Union, the United Kingdom has no alternative but to subscribe to the provisions of the EU Clinical Trials Directive. Nevertheless, the UK government is committed to re-negotiating the provisions of the directive to ensure that, in revised form, it is less burdensome, appropriately proportionate, and applied evenly across the European Union. At the same time, it will seek to ensure that patients' interests are safeguarded.

3. The National Institute for Health Research (NIHR) is developing metrics that will allow it to monitor the time taken for regulatory and governance approvals. The research charity, Cancer Research UK, estimates that in 2009 the time between its award of a grant to conduct a trial and the entry of the first patient averaged 631 days. The NIHR seeks for this to come down to 70 days. NHS hospitals failing to meet this requirement will face financial penalties.

Britain has a long and proud history of health research. The regulatory and governance arrangements instituted over the past 30 years have seriously eroded its historical position. The measures recently enacted, as well as those planned for the near future, should allow the United Kingdom to regain its rightful place in this endeavour (Rawlins, 2011).

REFERENCES

Academy of Medical Sciences. 2011. *A new pathway for the regulation and governance of health research*. London: Academy of Medical Sciences.

Rawlins, M. 2011. A new era for UK medical research? *Lancet* 377:190-193.

Appendix J

Discussion Paper[1]

Novel Ways to Get Good Trial Data: The UK Experience

Tom MacDonald, Isla Mackenzie, and Li Wei
Medical Research Institute of Dundee[2]

INTRODUCTION

Traditional randomised clinical trials are very expensive and time-consuming and often have poor external validity (Ware and Hamel, 2011). The challenge for modern medicine is to find ways of producing good-quality evidence with good external validity and to do so more efficiently, with less bureaucracy, more expeditiously, and above all less expensively than we have done in the past. To achieve these goals seems daunting at first but most of us work in organisations that already have amazing infrastructures that can be harnessed for research.

This paper will use the example of the United Kingdom (UK) National Health Service (NHS) but the methods are likely to be generalisable to other health care systems and health maintenance organisations.

The UK NHS is an organisation that has 61 million subjects about which everything is known (at least theoretically). These patients are

---

[1] The views expressed in this discussion paper are those of the authors and not necessarily of the authors' organizations or of the Institute of Medicine. The paper is intended to help inform and stimulate discussion. It has not been subjected to the review procedures of the Institute of Medicine and is not a report of the Institute of Medicine or of the National Research Council.

[2] Participants in the activities of the IOM Forum on Drug Discovery, Development, and Translation. This discussion paper is based on a submission to the Forum's November 2011 workshop, Envisioning a Transformed Clinical Trials Enterprise in the United States: Establishing an Agenda for 2020, to inform the workshop discussions surrounding international case studies in the area of clinical research transformation.

treated from cradle to grave in a system that is free at the point of delivery. So, there are data on all drug treatments (both prescribed and dispensed), all physician visits, all comorbidities, all laboratory tests, all hospitalisations, and all certified causes of deaths. In addition, there are data about ancestors and offspring and a lot of other detail about habits, social deprivation, etc. When asked in surveys, the public appears to support the use of these data to inform about the effectiveness and safety of medicines (Mackenzie et al., 2012).

The NHS in Scotland has traditionally had good record-linkage abilities due to far-sighted public health physicians in the 1960s (Kendrick, undated, 1997). This system has been utilised for observational research such as pharmacovigilance (Evans and MacDonald, 1999) and to develop clinical disease registers and managed clinical networks (Morris et al., 1997), but more recently record-linkage has been seen as an accurate way to track the outcomes of subjects randomised in clinical trials (Ford et al., 2007; West of Scotland Coronary Prevention Study Group, 1995).

RANDOMISING PATIENTS: STREAMLINED STUDIES

Randomising patients to different treatments within the NHS and using record-linkage to track outcomes is the concept behind the "streamlined study." Such studies can be double-blind with subjects being provided with masked investigational medicinal products (IMPs) or, if better external validity is required, internal validity can be traded by using open designs. The Febuxostat versus Allopurinol Streamlined Trial (FAST) study, which is running in the United Kingdom and Denmark, is an example of a streamlined study in which IMPs are provided to patients by mail. Follow-up is by a composite of e-mail, phone calls, family doctors, and record-linkage to hospitalisation and deaths.[3] Blinding the endpoints of this type of study (which are unlikely to be influenced by the patient's knowledge of what they are taking) results in the Prospective, Randomised, Open, Blinded Endpoint or PROBE design (Hansson et al., 1992). Of course, the ultimate "randomised effectiveness" study simply randomises therapy, which is then prescribed and compared to normal care prescribing. One such study, the Standard Care versus Celecoxib Outcome Trial (SCOT), is currently running in the United Kingdom, Denmark, and the Netherlands.[4] These "naturalistic" designs most closely mimic usual care and are designed to inform about the safety and effec-

---

[3] For more information on the FAST study, visit http://www.ukctg.nihr.ac.uk/trialdetails/ISRCTN72443728.

[4] For more information on the SCOT study, visit http://clinicaltrials.gov/ct2/show/NCT00447759.

tiveness of medicines and can help policy makers decide whether these medicines should be reimbursed.

The use of this type of trial design used specifically for post-approval safety research has recently been reviewed (Reynolds et al., 2011). Only 13 studies of this type of design were identified in this review, so these studies do not have an extensive track record. However, the authors concluded that this type of design has demonstrated utility for comparative research of medicines and vaccines.

University/NHS Sponsorship

There have been calls for studies of medicines to be run independently from the pharmaceutical industry (Steinbrook and Kassirer, 2010). In Europe, the study sponsor is the legal entity responsible for the conduct of a study and is independent of the study funder. We believe that academic and/or NHS sponsorship is the best way to carry out independent research on medicines and this is the mechanism under which we carry out this research, such as the SCOT and FAST trials (MacDonald et al., 2010).

PROS AND CONS OF STREAMLINED STUDIES

Streamlined studies make use of information technology (IT) to assist with the identification and invitation of patients to participate. In the case of the NHS, individual primary care physician practices can be recruited and contracted. These practices then allow electronic searches of their practice records to identify subjects who meet the study entry criteria. A list of potentially suitable subjects is scrutinised by the primary care physicians to remove subjects who they deem unsuitable to be contacted. The final list is then used to send letters to these subjects (the text of which is preapproved by the ethics committee) on practice notepaper and signed by the patient's doctor. A study patient information sheet is enclosed with this letter. Those patients who reply and who express willingness to be considered for study inclusion are then contacted by the study research nurse who takes consent, formally screens them using an electronic case report form, and randomises them using an interactive voice recognition system or online randomisation tool.

The benefit of using such a system is that large populations of patients who meet the inclusion and exclusion criteria for a study can be screened efficiently and invited to participate. Thus, in the SCOT study, for example, more than 630 family practices, representing a total population in excess of 4 million patients, have signed research contracts and had their records electronically searched to identify suitable study subjects. This is a highly efficient way to screen large populations.

The follow-up of subjects is also efficient as all hospitalisations and deaths are recorded centrally in the United Kingdom, so subjects can be efficiently tracked by record-linkage. Secure, study-specific web portals allow family physicians and study staff to report adverse events, adjust medication, track laboratory results, etc. NHS records of hospitalisations suspected of being endpoints can be retrieved, scanned into portable document format, redacted where necessary, and abstracted to forms to allow endpoint committee adjudication. Such adjudication is also done using remote secure systems that allow geographically diverse end-point committee members to interact efficiently.

These electronic systems allow efficiencies that reduce the overall costs of research. It seems to be even better in Denmark, where prescribing records are collated centrally along with hospitalisation and mortality data and where the population seems to welcome, and even expect, electronic records to be used for research purposes. However, these electronic systems do not solve all study problems.

Bureaucracy

The bureaucratic processes of obtaining multiple consents and approvals required to carry out clinical research are not diminished by such study designs (Duley et al., 2008; McMahon et al., 2009). This article is not the place to rehearse these issues. Suffice it to say that the UK Academy of Medical Sciences has produced a report for the UK government on this matter that has made a number of recommendations aimed at reducing this burden of bureaucracy (The Academy of Medical Sciences, 2011). (See also the Institute of Medicine discussion paper by Sir Michael Rawlins, *Health Research as a Public Good*, 2012.)

Engaging Patients in Research

A major hurdle facing streamlined studies (as well as other clinical studies) is how to engage patients in the health research agenda. While we can efficiently identify suitable subjects electronically based on eligibility criteria, for every 100 patients written to, our experience is that an average of only 14 subjects are randomised. The dominant reason for this is that most patients do not reply to letters of invitation written to them by their family physicians. In inner-city practices in the United Kingdom, 70 percent or more of subjects do not reply at all. In rural practices, we get more replies and more positive replies, perhaps because patients have closer relationships with their family doctors in the rural setting. However, while electronically searching family physician records provides a way of writing to large cohorts of suitable patients, it does not solve the problem of how to engage patients in research and enhance recruitment. Several reviews have addressed this issue (Caldwell et al., 2010; Treweek et al., 2010). Despite trying numerous initiatives, we have not yet found a good solution to this problem (see Box 1 and Mackenzie et al., 2010). Cracking this difficult nut will require effort.

Paying Patients?

We have recently received ethical committee approval for a study to formally evaluate the effect of paying patients an incentive of £100 (about $150) to participate in clinical trials. This method has some evidence base (Halpern et al., 2004; Martinson et al., 2000) and appears to be common practice in the United States (Dickert et al., 2002). Perhaps this could provide a solution both to recruiting more subjects and to recruiting subjects who are more representative of the population at large.

Event Rates

Clinical outcome trials are designed to include subjects who are likely to experience outcome events. Even for a composite outcome such as hospitalisation for myocardial infarction, cerebrovascular accident, or vascular death, the expected event rate may only be 1 to 2 percent per year even in an "at-risk" older population. A problem that bedevils trialists is that the patients enrolled into studies often have event rates lower than expected. There are many potential explanations for this phenomenon but one explanation is that patients who respond positively to letters of invitation to participate are those who have an interest in their health and thus exhibit good heath behaviour and are therefore at lower risk of events. Subjects with poor health behaviour are less likely to participate. Clearly, trials of younger patients with few risk factors could not feasibly examine outcome events as these studies would have to be unfeasibly large or long, or both, to generate sufficient events. Because of this, streamlined studies have to limit recruitment to older subjects preferably with additional risk factors in order to limit the size and duration of the trial to reasonable parameters. As with all studies that restrict inclusion of subjects, the generalisability, or external validity, of such studies is reduced by such restrictions. However, even when entry is restricted to high-risk and older age groups, event rates can be low. The very elderly and the socially deprived are underrepresented in clinical trials. Part of the engagement of the public in research must be to target these groups and stress how important it is that they are included.

Post-Randomisation Control

A potential criticism of streamlined studies is that there is relatively little patient contact post-randomisation. While a lack of scheduled patient visits reduces dramatically the costs of follow-up, an argument can be made that it also results in a loss of post-randomisation "control" of the study. Usually, subjects in randomised trials are "encouraged" to persist with randomised medication until the end of the trial. In streamlined studies (by design), persistence with medication more closely resembles normal care. Thus, subjects may be more likely to switch randomised medication. The effect of this is that streamlined studies become more "observational" with time. For superiority studies where the primary analysis is the "intention to treat" population, switching of medication post-randomisation will dilute the observed efficacy. However, the result will be more informative of the likely effectiveness of such an intervention being introduced into normal care. Clearly, such clinical effectiveness is the metric that drives decisions about cost-effectiveness. For non-inferiority designs in which the primary outcome of interest is a per-protocol analysis, switching therapy post-randomisation results in subjects being censored at the point of switching with a resulting reduction in the person-years exposure to medication and thus reduced power of the study. Streamlined studies need to take this factor into account in the design stage and over-recruit subjects to compensate for this effect. In addition, these studies should prospectively plan to carry out an observational type of analysis by treatment taken at the time of an event as a supporting post hoc analysis. Such analyses need to be developed.

ALTERNATIVES TO RANDOMISING PATIENTS INTO STREAMLINED STUDIES

Whilst streamlined studies have many advantages, they are not a perfect solution to getting good data quickly and inexpensively. For this reason we have explored other methods of evaluating treatments.

Randomising Family Practice Prescribing or Cluster Randomisation

In the United Kingdom, family practices invariably adopt a limited list or practice formulary of medications to which their practice computer systems default when they prescribe. These formularies are often derived from regional formularies which in turn are derived from the recommendations of bodies such as the Scottish Medicines Consortium (SMC)[5] or the National Institute for Clinical Excellence (NICE).[6]

---

[5] For more information on the SMC, visit http://www.scottishmedicines.org.uk/Home.

[6] For more information on NICE, visit http://www.nice.org.uk.

There are 15,158 practices in the UK NHS. If half of even a small proportion of these used one medication for a particular indication and the other half used a different medication, then a cluster randomised design would produce excellent outcome data very quickly as the sheer numbers involved would allow studies of even quite rare conditions to be done. This method provides a framework for the pragmatic evaluation of the comparative effectiveness of medications (Maclure, 2009), and we have found that such designs are supported by the public (Mackenzie et al., 2012).

One such study is already under way as a pilot in the United Kingdom. This is a British Hypertension Society Research Network study titled A Randomised Policy Trial to Evaluate the Optimal Policy Diuretic for the Treatment of Hypertension. This trial seeks to formally evaluate the new proposals from NICE to change diuretic therapy for hypertension in the United Kingdom from bendroflumethiazide to chlortalidone or indapamide,[7] guidance which has been criticised for having a poor evidence base (Brown et al., 2012).

How Randomising Practice Formulary Studies Are Done

The way these studies work is that practices agree to participate and are then randomly allocated a drug (or treatment strategy) to implement. Each practice writes to all patients affected by this formulary change to tell them that the practice has decided to change (or not to change) their formulary first-choice drug for the purposes of aiding the evaluation to determine which drug is the better treatment. Patients are informed that this change will be evaluated and that their anonymised data will be used in this evaluation. Patients are offered the opportunity to opt out of the change of drug or to opt out of their anonymised data being used in the evaluation.

The pilot phase of the current diuretic study seeks to determine the workload generated to practices by writing to patients and dealing with feedback and potential opt-outs. Clearly, the level of remuneration required by practices will depend on this workload. However, the majority of general practitioners surveyed are supportive of this type of evaluation, and we believe that the majority of patients also support the NHS evaluation of drugs used in the NHS (Mackenzie et al., 2012).

Recently, the UK government has announced an initiative suggesting that everyone in the NHS should contribute to research and become research patients.[8] Such an initiative will hopefully support this type of

---

[7] For the NICE proposal on changing diuretic therapy for hypertension in the United Kingdom, visit http://guidance.nice.org.uk.

[8] For more information on the UK government's announcement, visit http://www.bbc.co.uk/news/uk-16026827.

trial design, in which the NHS evaluates the medicines the NHS uses (Mackenzie et al., 2012).

Ethical Considerations

Ethical issues concerning cluster randomised trial designs have been debated but no clear consensus has been reached (Taljaard et al., 2009). When asked about the ethics of cluster-randomising new practice guidelines that were drawn up based on opinion versus previous guidelines, most panelists at a recent conference in Ottawa were of the view that it would be unethical not to do such an evaluation (International Consensus Conference, 2011). Such randomised policy designs and variants have long been promoted by Malcolm Maclure and others (Maclure et al., 2007). Their widespread use would enable us to know which drug-prescribing policies are good or bad. At present, we never know.

Evaluating New Medicines

Family practice–based cluster randomised studies could provide the framework to study the effectiveness of newly licensed therapies. Mechanisms to limit the use of novel drugs exist worldwide because of financial constraints on drug budgets. Such policies make it very difficult for manufacturers of novel therapies to collect observational, postmarketing data on safety and effectiveness. However, if half of a large group of participating practices changed their prescribing to a novel medicine from the standard therapy, then half of the population would enjoy the latest therapy at no cost to the NHS, as the pharmaceutical industry would provide such study medication free (or reimburse the NHS for its cost). Such a system provides a low-cost framework to judge the effectiveness and safety of novel therapies expeditiously. Since clinical effectiveness is the principal driver of cost-effectiveness, such a system would provide the data to support the widespread introduction (or not) of new treatments.

Advantages of Cluster Randomising Practice Formularies

A major advantage of cluster randomisation is that the costs and bureaucracy of doing these studies are minimal. A feature of the design of these trials means that the analyses are done using anonymised data. This means that the trial sponsor has no way of determining which patients experience serious adverse events. However, family doctors can still report such events directly to the regulatory authorities in an anonymous fashion.

Discussions have been held with the UK Medicines and Healthcare products Regulatory Agency (MHRA) as to the requirement of such studies to obtain clinical trial authorisation. The ruling at present is that the particular diuretic comparison study described above is not within the scope of the clinical trials directive as, although practices are randomised, individual patients still have the ability to determine their own treatment (M. Ward & E. Godfrey, MHRA, personal communication). It is probable that similar designs of other drug comparisons using such cluster randomisation would be regarded in the same way.

Design variants of randomising practice policies might be appropriate if, for example, the purpose of the evaluation were to determine the effectiveness of a new therapy thought to be beneficial when added to existing therapy. Designed delay studies (sometimes known as the stepped wedge design) might be judged ethically appropriate in such instances, especially where the implementation of such a new prescribing policy is limited by resource constraints. Such designs gradually introduce policy "randomly." For example, if 100 practices were studied, a few would start with the new policy in the first month, a few in the second month, and so on, until all 100 practices had introduced the new policy. The beauty of such a system is that it produces data with excellent external validity and everyone gets the new policy over the course of the study.

New European legislation on the post-licensing risk management of novel marketed medicines will place a greater onus on manufacturers to gather postmarketing data on their products (Waller, 2011). This will stimulate better methods of data collection post-licensing and NICE and the SMC will stimulate the need for better comparative-effectiveness data.

Other Trial Designs

Good-quality prospective safety data can be collected directly from patients, as was shown in a recent prospective follow-up study of subjects vaccinated against the H1N1 virus (Mackenzie et al., 2011). Here, subjects being vaccinated responded to posters and volunteered to be followed up by e-mail, text message, or telephone. This system worked well and has stimulated other study designs that could be adapted. An example is the British Hypertension Society Research Network Treatment In the Morning versus Evening (TIME) study.[9] This study advertises to potential participants who are willing to log on, consent, and be randomised in taking their antihypertensive medication in the morning or the evening. Patients are followed up by regular e-mails and record-linkage. One can envision a future scenario in which patients are recruited on the Internet, screened online, and agree to their physician giving assent, then are randomized,

---

[9] For more information on the TIME study, see www.demo.timestudy.co.uk for a demonstration. The full site is www.timestudy.co.uk.

mailed medication, and followed up by e-mail, with their own physician or record-linkage providing outcome data. Investigator training in Good Clinical Practice and trial startup training can be provided by webinars to defray the cost of the usual face-to-face training. Table 1 summarizes the pros and cons of each of the trial designs discussed above.

CONCLUSION

Most of the design concepts presented here have been implemented by us at least into the pilot phase. Not everyone will agree with the ethical approach, or the robustness or feasibility of these designs, but experience will teach us how to adapt these concepts to improve the cost-effectiveness of obtaining high-quality data. We have found that the public are largely supportive of initiatives to improve the safety and effectiveness of medicines (Mackenzie et al., 2012). As a society we need to continue to think up better ways to acquire high-quality data to enhance and make health care delivery more efficient.

REFERENCES

Academy of Medical Sciences. 2011. *A new pathway for the regulation and governance of health research.* http://www.acmedsci.ac.uk/p47prid88.html (accessed January 16, 2012).

Brown, M. J., J. K. Cruickshank, and T. M. Macdonald. 2012. Navigating the shoals in hypertension: Discovery and guidance. *British Medical Journal* 344:d8218, doi:10.1136/bmj.d8218.

Caldwell, P. H., S. Hamilton, A. Tan, and J. C. Craig. 2010. Strategies for increasing recruitment to randomised controlled trials: Systematic review. *PLoS Med* 7(11):e1000368.

Dickert, N., E. Emanuel, and C. Grady. 2002. Paying research subjects: An analysis of current policies. *Annals of Internal Medicine* 136:368-373.

Duley, L., K. Antman, J. Arena, A. Avezum, M. Blumenthal, J. Bosch, S. Chrolavicius, T. Li, S. Ounpuu, A. C. Perez, P. Sleight, R. Svard, R. Temple, Y. Tsouderous, C. Yunis, and S. Yusuf. 2008. Specific barriers to the conduct of randomized trials. *Clinical Trials* 5:40-48.

Evans, J. M. M., and T. M. MacDonald. 1999. Record-linkage for pharmacovigilance in Scotland. *British Journal of Clinical Pharmacology* 47:105-110.

Ford, I., H. Murray, C. J. Packard, J. Shepherd, P. W. Macfarlane, S. M. Cobbe (West of Scotland Coronary Prevention Study Group). 2007. Long-term follow-up of the West of Scotland Coronary Prevention Study. *New England Journal of Medicine* 357:1477-1486.

Halpern, S. D., J. H. Karlawish, D. Casarett, J. A. Berlin, and D. A. Asch. 2004. Empirical assessment of whether moderate payments are undue or unjust inducements for participation in clinical trials. *Archives of Internal Medicine* 164:801-803.

Hansson, L., T. Hedner, and B. Dahlof. 1992. Prospective randomised open blinded endpoint (PROBE) study. A novel design for intervention trials. *Blood Pressure* 1:113-119.

International Consensus Conference to Generate Ethics Guidelines for Cluster Randomized Trials. 2011. Ottawa, Ontario, November 28-30.

Kendrick, S. Undated. *The Scottish record linkage system.* http://www.isdscotland.org/Products-and-Services/Medical-Record-Linkage/Files-for-upload/The_Scottish_Record_Linkage_ System.doc (accessed January 9, 2012).

Kendrick, S. 1997. Chapter 10: The development of record linkage in Scotland. *Record Linkage Techniques.* www.fcsm.gov/working-papers/skendrick.pdf (accessed January 9, 2012).

MacDonald, T., C. Hawkey, and I. Ford. 2010. Academic sponsorship. Time to treat as independent. *British Medical Journal* 341, doi:10.1136/bmj.c6837.

Mackenzie, I. S., L. Wei, D. Rutherford, E. A. Findlay, W. Saywood, M. K. Campbell, and T. M. MacDonald. 2010. Promoting public understanding of randomised clinical trials using the media: The "Get Randomised" campaign. *British Journal of Clinical Pharmacology* 69:128-135.

Mackenzie, I. S., T. M. Macdonald, S. Shakir, M. Dryburgh, B. J. Mantay, P. McDonnell, and D. Layton. 2011. Influenza H1N1 (swine flu) vaccination: A safety surveillance feasibility study using self-reporting of serious adverse events and pregnancy outcomes. *British Journal of Clinical Pharmacology* (Nov 15), doi:10.1111/j.1365-2125.2011.04142.x [Epub ahead of print].

Mackenzie, I. S., L. Wei, K. R. Paterson, and T. M. MacDonald. 2012. Cluster randomised trials of prescription medicines or prescribing policy—public and general practitioner opinions in Scotland. *British Journal of Clinical Pharmacology* (Jan 30), doi: 10.1111/j.1365-2125.2012.04195.x [Epub ahead of print].

Maclure, M. 2009. Explaining pragmatic trials to pragmatic policy-makers. *Canadian Medical Association Journal* 180:1001-1003.

Maclure, M., B. Carleton, and S. Schneeweiss. 2007. Designed delays versus rigorous pragmatic trials: Lower carat gold standards can produce relevant drug evaluations. *Medical Care* 45(10 Suppl 2):S44-S49.

Martinson, B. C., D. Lazovich, H. A. Lando, C. L. Perry, P. G. McGovern, and R. G. Boyle. 2000. Effectiveness of monetary incentives for recruiting adolescents to an intervention trial to reduce smoking. *Preventive Medicine* 31:706-713.

McMahon, A. D., D. I. Conway, T. M. Macdonald, and G. T. McInnes. The unintended consequences of clinical trials regulations. 2009. *PLoS Med* 3(11):e1000131.

Morris, A. D., D. I. R. Boyle, R. McAlpine, A. Emslie-Smith, R. T. Jung, R. W. Newton, and T. M. MacDonald. 1997. The Diabetes Audit and Research in Tayside Scotland (DARTS) study: Electronic record linkage to create a diabetes register. *British Medical Journal* 315:524-528.

Reynolds, R. F., J. A. Lem, N. M. Gatto, and S. M. Eng. 2011. Is the large simple trial design used for comparative, post-approval safety research? A review of a clinical trials registry and the published literature. *Drug Safety* 34:799-820.

Steinbrook, R., and J. P. Kassirer. 2010. Data availability for industry sponsored trials: What should medical journals require? *British Medical Journal* 341, doi:10.1136/bmj.c5391.

Taljaard, M., C. Weijer, J. M. Grimshaw, J. B. Brown, A. Binik, R. Boruch, J. C. Brehaut, S. H. Chaudhry, M. P. Eccles, A. McRae, R. Saginur, M. Zwarenstein, and A. Donner. 2009. Ethical and policy issues in cluster randomized trials: Rationale and design of a mixed methods research study. *Trials* 10:61, doi:10.1186/1745-6215-10-61.

Treweek, S., M. Pitkethly, J. Cook, M. Kjeldstrøm, T. Taskila, M. Johansen, F. Sullivan, S. Wilson, C. Jackson, R. Jones, and E. Mitchell. Strategies to improve recruitment to randomised controlled trials. 2010. *Cochrane Database Syst Rev* (4):MR000013.

Waller, P. 2011. Getting to grips with the new European Union pharmacovigilance legislation. *Pharmacoepidemiology and Drug Safety* 20:544-549, doi:10.1002/pds.2119.

Ware, J. H., and M. B. Hamel. 2011. Pragmatic trials—guides to better patient care? *New England Journal of Medicine* 364:1685-1687.

West of Scotland Coronary Prevention Study Group. 1995. Computerised record linkage: Compared with traditional patient follow-up methods in clinical trials and illustrated in a prospective epidemiological study. *Journal of Clinical Epidemiology* 48:1441-1452.

BOX 1
Patient Recruitment/Public Engagement Initiatives
That Have Not Worked in Our Experience

- Television campaigns aimed at engaging patients (Mackenzie et al., 2010)
  — Very costly, raised awareness but did not change recruitment

- Advertisements in local and national newspapers and local radio
  — Costly, ineffective, and attracted small numbers of mostly unsuitable subjects

- Publicity for clinical trials in local newspaper articles
  — Attracted mostly unsuitable subjects

- Study-specific websites (i.e., http://www.scottrial.co.uk/)
  — Did not attract study subjects

- Multiple revisions of patient letters from family doctors
  — Did not affect patient response rate
  — Follow-up letters to non-responders were not effective

- Postage options
  — Normal, first-class, registered/courier delivery made no difference in patient response rate

- Publicised open public meetings to discuss clinical research with suitable patients also invited on an individual basis by physicians (including general talks of interest, i.e., a physiotherapist discussing exercises for arthritis
  — Public meetings did not attract patients

TABLE 1 Advantages and Disadvantages of Individual Study Designs Discussed in This Paper

STUDY TYPE	ADVANTAGES	DISADVANTAGES
Streamlined trials	• Population-based so potentially good external validity • Large populations searched • Only suitable subjects invited • Reflects normal care • Reduced cost	• Self-selected "healthier" subjects sign up so external validity is not perfect • ~ 50% of practices do not participate • Few subjects accept • Become "observational" rapidly • Similar bureaucracy
Cluster randomised trials	• Reduced bureaucracy • Large populations studied efficiently • Most patients participate • No individual patient consent • Inexpensive, efficient, & quick • Treatments prescribed • Record-linkage outcomes • Do not (usually) need a clinical trials authorisation	• Only anonymous data retrieved • Reduced statistical power from cluster design • Opt-out patients may bias study • Requires practices to consent • Requires efficient electronic tracking of anonymous subjects • Only suitable for products with a marketing authorisation. May be criticised as "seeding studies" • End-point validation required • Not suitable for all health outcome studies
Prospective observational follow-up studies	• Consented subjects • Patient-reported outcomes • Able to contact patients • Large cohorts & frequent e-mail contact • Patients self-selected & more likely to take part in other research • Observes normal care	• Reduced data privacy issues • Outcomes need to be validated (via family doctor) and coded • Ease of capture of further data • IT and clinical support resource issues • May not be representative of the population • Not randomised
Internet-only randomised trials of drug therapy	• Theoretically feasible • Inexpensive • Patient-driven recruitment • Recruited by targeted advertising (i.e. doctor surgeries) • Internet only • Less field-based manpower required • Single-centre studies	• Must comply with clinical trials legislation • Data-quality assurance required • Require family doctor assent • Need to engage public in research agenda to maximize utility • Requires Internet access and IT-literate subjects • More IT and office-based clinical staff • Bureaucracy may still be significant

Appendix K

IOM Staff Paper

Context and Glossary of Select Terms Associated with the Clinical Trials Enterprise

Rebecca English
Institute of Medicine, Forum on Drug Discovery,
Development, and Translation

CONTEXT

The following is a glossary of clinical research terms drawn from planning discussions and conversations that took place at the November 2011 workshop summarized in this report. These definitions were not formally presented at the workshop but have been compiled retrospectively by Institute of Medicine (IOM) staff to clarify some of the terms used at the workshop. The glossary was developed to provide greater background information to the reader who may be unfamiliar with the terms but is not intended to be an exhaustive or complete list of terms relevant to the clinical trials enterprise. These are practical working definitions to help the reader understand the terms used.

All clinical trials are designed to answer one or more specific questions. They can vary by the study population chosen (number of subjects, as well as criteria to enter the study) and the type of question(s) posed. For example, clinical trials to gain U.S. Food and Drug Administration (FDA) approval for a new drug are designed to show its safety and efficacy over the course of a specified period of time—traditionally using a randomized controlled clinical trial design (RCT) (IOM, 2010a). These trials seek to answer narrowly defined questions related to safety and efficacy in a carefully selected group of study participants most likely to experience the intended effects of the drug. Clinical trials conducted without the goal of regulatory approval might test a drug or intervention in a diverse group of study participants, include a longer time frame for follow-up of study subjects, and address a broader set of questions.

Although RCTs, the primary focus of the Forum's workshop series on clinical trials, will continue to play an important role in the development of new drugs and therapies, many believe the approach is not always feasible, ethical, or practical to answer the wide array of research questions facing the nation today. The scientific value of RCTs is well established, but the high cost and time commitment required for these studies, combined with the often limited applicability of results to patient populations that differ from those in the original study, can disassociate this type of research from the reality of medical practice. A primary theme of the workshop is the need to bridge the divide between clinical research and clinical practice— i.e., to effectively bring clinical research into the community. Doing so would involve partnerships among researchers, physicians, and patients and facilitate the development of studies focused on answering meaningful questions for clinical practice, which in turn could inform the development of new, targeted therapies for the changing health needs of the population.

Workshop participants discussed a broad range of research methods that would engage patients and clinicians and go beyond determinations of efficacy (i.e., can it work under ideal circumstances?) to evaluate clinical effectiveness (i.e., can it work in real world, clinical practice settings?). It was noted at the workshop that the full battery of clinical research methods will be necessary to improve our understanding of the questions that emerge through the lifecycle of a medical product. For instance, Figure 1 suggests a timeline of medical products research and the corresponding development of various types of evidence.

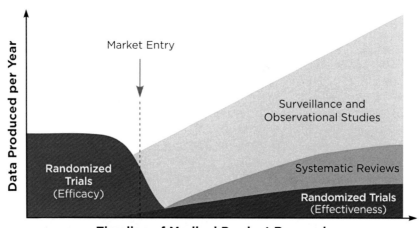

FIGURE 1 Evidence development in the learning health system over the course of a medical product's lifetime.
SOURCE: IOM, 2010b. *Redesigning the Clinical Effectiveness Research Paradigm.*

GLOSSARY

Adaptive trial design: experimental study design in which the treatment allocation ratio of an RCT is altered based on a prespecified plan defining prescribed changes to study end points, and other criteria, over the course of the study based on collected data and treatment responses of prior participants. Bayesian or Frequentist analyses are based on the accumulated treatment responses of prior participants and used to inform adaptive designs by assessing the probability or frequency, respectively, with which an event of interest occurs (e.g., positive response to a particular treatment) (IOM, 2010b).

Clinical effectiveness research: a type of research that builds on safety and efficacy determinations necessary for regulatory approval to develop research results to guide the delivery of appropriate care to individual patients (IOM, 2010b). Clinical effectiveness research includes a broad range of research designs and data sources—including post-marketing data for medical products.

Clinical trial: a medical research study in humans to evaluate the effects of one or more interventions/treatments. Clinical trials typically evaluate the effects of an intervention by comparing the outcomes of a group receiving the intervention and a group receiving standard care (when there is no standard of care, a placebo is traditionally used). Data on adverse events are typically collected systematically during such trials. Clinical trials (also called "research studies") are used to determine whether new drugs or treatments are safe and effective. See definitions below of randomized controlled clinical trials and non-randomized clinical trials for information on the merits of each design.

Clinical trials enterprise (CTE): a broad term that encompasses the full spectrum of clinical trials and their applications. The CTE includes the processes, institutions, and individuals that eventually apply clinical trial findings to patient care.

ClinicalTrials.gov: a publicly funded and available registry (http://clinicaltrials.gov/) of completed and ongoing clinical trials. The database, which was mandated in the Food and Drug Administration Modernization Act (FDAMA) of 1997, is intended to serve as a centralized information source for clinical trials including studies on products regulated by FDA. The registry was developed in 2000, is administered by the NIH's National Library of Medicine (NLM), and includes federally and privately supported clinical trials. Study sponsors are responsible for submitting timely and accurate information to ClinicalTrials.gov about their trials before the trial is started, while it is ongoing (should there be changes), and after the trial is completed. The number of trials registered increased substantially in 2005 as a result of a requirement by the International Committee of Medical Journal Editors (ICMJE) that studies published in ICMJE-associated journals be registered on ClinicalTrials.gov or another equivalent publicly available trial registry.

Cluster Randomized Controlled Trial: an experimental study design in which groups (e.g., individuals or patients from entire clinics, schools, communities, or physician practices), instead of individuals, are randomized to a particular treatment or study arm. This design is useful for a wide array of clinical effectiveness topics and may be required in situations in which individual randomization is not feasible. (IOM, 2010b). For an example of physician practices in the UK participating in a cluster randomized controlled trial, see the Discussion Paper in Appendix J, *Novel Ways to Get Good Trial Data: the UK Experience.*

Continuous improvement: quality improvement activities, typically conducted by health care delivery organizations, to assess processes of providing care to meet patient needs. These activities usually compare the relative effectiveness of delivering existing approved therapies or diagnostics. IOM reports in 2000 and 2001 found that most medical errors resulted from faulty processes and systems, not individuals. Quality improvement efforts to identify and correct errors and inefficiencies in the processes of delivering patient care have become common practice within health care delivery organizations. Today, the concept of continuous improvement in health care includes more than just measurements of quality and could also incorporate innovation and a strong scientific foundation to inform improvement efforts. Several workshop participants suggested that to pursue the goal of further integrating clinical research and practice, policy change or clarification be taken up that would expressly permit inclusion of routine evidence generation activities of health care organizations that pose no more than a minimal risk to patients under the concept of continuous improvement activities, which would have the effect of exempting these activities from the traditional regulatory framework applied to experimental research activities (e.g., Common Rule, HIPAA). They noted that incorporating low-risk research into the concept of continuous improvement could improve the ability of health care systems to engage in research efforts. For a discussion of the distinctions between continuous improvement—including quality and clinical effectiveness assessments—and human subjects research that requires formal oversight by an Institutional Review Board (IRB), see Selker et al., 2011.

Coverage with Evidence Development (CED): an insurance coverage and simultaneous evidence-development strategy under which the Centers for Medicare and Medicaid Services (CMS) issues a National Coverage Determination (NCD) requiring, as a condition of paying for a particular treatment under federal programs, prospective collection of additional patient data to supplement standard claims data. Under a CED decision, in order for Medicare to pay for a particular treatment patients must agree to participate in a clinical trial or registry to further evaluate the risks and benefits of that product. Although the term "coverage with evidence development" was first coined in a draft guidance issued by the CMS in April 2005, the policy of linking Medicare coverage with clinical research began in 1995 (Tunis and Pearson, 2006).

Direct-to-patient trial: a new research approach that recruits, administers therapeutics, and monitors clinical trial participants via the internet. Also called a "virtual" clinical trial, this could result in faster clinical trials as the potentially eligible patient population includes anyone with internet access—as opposed to the current model that relies on recruiting patients who live in close proximity to clinical trial sites. Trial sponsors could also realize lower clinical trial costs using this model because individual "brick and mortar" trial sites would not need to be set up across the country. The first FDA approved "virtual" clinical trial is being conducted by Pfizer to evaluate the safety and efficacy of an overactive bladder drug.

Electronic data capture (EDC): a technological tool that facilitates the collection of data electronically from clinical trial sites. EDC can reduce errors in data sent from trial sites to the coordinating center and trial sponsor and can help make clinical trial results available faster (Kush, 2006). Use of EDC in clinical trials was discussed during the workshop by some participants who noted that other risk-management practices of clinical trial sponsors, such as having a monitor travel to a clinical trial site to compare hard copies of patient EHRs and EDC printouts instead of correlating this information from electronic archive systems, can nullify the originally intended efficiencies of EDC.

Electronic Health Record (EHR): an electronic tool that captures a wide range of information related to a patient's health, entered by health care providers in various settings, and aggregates the data to serve different needs. According to the Healthcare Information and Management Systems Society (HIMSS), an electronic health record is defined as a longitudinal electronic record of patient health information generated by one or more encounters in any care delivery setting. Included in this information are patient demographics, progress notes, problems, medications, vital signs, past medical history, immunizations, laboratory data, and radiology reports. The data in the EHR is used to generate a complete record of a clinical patient encounter, as well as supporting other care-related activities directly or indirectly via interface, including evidence-based decision support, quality management, and outcomes reporting. Beyond patient-specific medical data, EHRs include clinical decision support tools, computerized provider order entry systems, and e-prescribing systems (IOM, 2012). As discussed during the workshop, use of the EHR for clinical research purposes could play a key role in bridging the current divide between clinical research and practice.

Equipoise: the point at which a rational, informed person would not have a preference between the therapies in each arm of a trial (Lilford and Jackson, 1995). In clinical trials, the ethical concept of equipoise is satisfied when genuine physician and patient uncertainty exists as to the comparative benefits of the therapies in each treatment group of the trial. The concept and applicability of equipoise have been debated, as differences between the uncertainties and preferences of an individual (individual equipoise) and society (collective equipoise) can vary (Chard and Lilford, 1998).

Good Clinical Practice (GCP): an international ethical and scientific quality standard for designing, conducting, recording, and reporting trials that involve the participation of human subjects (ICH, 1996). Satisfying GCP requirements provides assurance that the data and reported results of the clinical trial are credible and accurate and that the rights, integrity, and confidentiality of trial subjects are protected (ICH, 1996). GCP guidelines are developed by the International Conference on Harmonisation of Technical Requirements for Registration of Pharmaceuticals for Human Use (ICH), which brings together regulatory authorities and pharmaceutical industry of Europe, Japan, and United States.

Non-randomized clinical trial: a clinical trial design in which patients are not assigned by chance to different treatment groups—instead the patient or his/her practitioner might choose her or his treatment group or be assigned to a group by a researcher. In either scenario, the assignment to a treatment group is not left to chance.

Observational study: a type of research in which the investigator observes the measure of interest and no interventions or treatments are provided as part of the study. Patient registries and EHRs are examples of data sources for an observational study. When it is not considered ethical or feasible to answer a research question using a controlled trial, an observational study could develop information to answer the research question or advance a hypothesis, which could, in turn, be tested by a future RCT. Because observational studies have less internal validity (i.e., greater opportunity for the introduction of bias in the study) than an RCT, the results are not always sufficient to base a decision to change medical practice. However, valuable information can be gathered through observational studies about the implementation and use of medical treatments in clinical practice. Because observational studies can feasibly collect data on large populations over a long period of time, they are the most reliable way to gather data on rare medical events.

Patient-centered outcomes research (PCOR): PCOR in the United States, being further developed and funded by the independent Patient-Centered Outcomes Research Institute (PCORI), aims to help people and their caregivers make informed health care decisions and allows their voice to be heard in assessing the value of health care options (PCORI, 2012). PCOR could involve clinical effectiveness research methods as well as head-to-head comparisons to evaluate the relative strengths and weaknesses of various interventions. PCOR is similar to what is called "patient-oriented research" in Canada's current strategy to improve health outcomes and enhance patient's health care experience based on translation of research outcomes into the health care system (see Discussion Paper in Appendix H for more information on the effort in Canada).

Protocol: an extensive "blueprint" for the clinical trial including the trial objective, design, methodology, and organization. Protocols are required to be submitted to the relevant institutions and organizations that provide ethical and regulatory approval for clinical trials. Protocol design plays a crucial role in the success of a trial as it outlines exactly what the trial will entail, the eligibility criteria for those who can participate, and the frequency of the procedures and treatments that trial participants will be expected to receive over the course of the study. In recent years, protocols have become more complex and demanding for clinical trial sites to implement. One study found that the number of unique procedures and the frequency of procedures per clinical trial protocol have increased at an annual rate of 6.5 percent and 8.7 percent, respectively, from 1999 to 2005 (Getz et al., 2008). Researchers found that over this same time period, study conduct performance worsened—patient recruitment and retention rates lowered, more amendments to the clinical trial protocol were initiated, and more serious adverse events were observed (Getz et al., 2008).

Randomized controlled clinical trial (RCT): an experimental study design in which patients are randomly allocated to treatment groups in a trial. Analysis estimates the size of difference in predefined outcomes, under ideal treatment conditions, between treatment groups. "Controlled" refers to the standard that allows experimental observations to the evaluated—the control group of patients receives standard treatment or placebo to provide the basis for comparing the effect of the experimental treatment given to the other group of patients. Randomly assigning patients to receive the intervention addresses concerns that known or unknown differences in intervention groups might affect the outcome of the trial. RCTs are characterized by a focus on efficacy, internal validity, maximal compliance with the assigned regimen (see definition of "protocol" above), and typically, complete patient follow up. When feasible and appropriate, trials are "double-blind"—i.e., both patients and trialists are unaware of treatment assignment throughout the study (IOM, 2010b). Not all clinical trials are randomized (see the above definition of non-randomized clinical trial).

REFERENCES

Chard, J. A. and R. J. Lilford. 1998. The use of equipoise in clinical trials. *Social Science & Medicine* 47(7):891-898.

ClinicalTrials.gov. http://clinicaltrials.gov/ct2/info/glossary.

Getz, K. A., J. Wenger, R. A. Campo, E. S. Sequine, and K. I. Kaitin. 2008. Assessing the impact of protocol design change on clinical trial performance. *American Journal of Therapeutics* 15(5): 450-457.

Institute of Medicine (IOM). 2010a. *Transforming clinical research in the United States: Challenges and opportunities. Workshop Summary.* Washington, DC: The National Academies Press.

IOM. 2010b. *Redesigning the clinical effectiveness research paradigm: Innovation and practice-based approaches. Workshop Summary.* Washington, DC: The National Academies Press.

IOM. 2012. *Health IT and patient safety: Building safer systems for better care.* Washington, DC: The National Academies Press.

International Conference on Harmonisation of Technical Requirements for Registration of Pharmaceuticals for Human Use (ICH). 1996. *Guidance for industry E6 good clinical practice: Consolidated guidance.* http://www.fda.gov/Drugs/GuidanceCompliance RegulatoryInformation/Guidances/ucm065004.htm (accessed February 15, 2012).

Kush, R. 2006. Electronic data capture—pros and cons. *BioExecutive International* 2(6):S48-S52.

Patient-Centered Outcomes Research Institutes (PCORI). 2012. *Patient-Centered Outcomes Research.* http://www.pcori.org/patient-centered-outcomes-research/ (accessed April 9, 2012).

Selker, H., C. Grossman, A. Adams, D. Goldmann, C. Dezii, G. Meyer, V. Roger, L. Savitz, and R. Platt. 2011. *The common rule and continuous improvement in health care: A learning health system perspective.* Discussion Paper, Institute of Medicine, Washington, DC. http://www.iom.edu/Global/Perspectives/2012/CommonRule.aspx (accessed February 3, 2012).

Tunis, S. R. and S. D. Pearson. 2006. Coverage options for promising technologies: Medicare's coverage with evidence development. *Health Affairs* 25(5):1218-1230.